ᴀCKNOWLEDGMENTS

Ginger Ann Walker - Author and Publisher

Garrett Williams - Editor and Researcher

Nancy Adams Arnold - Layout Design and Production

First Edition 2020

Printed and bound in the United States of America.

Available through amazon.com and bookstores

ISBN: 9781087909578 (Paperback)

Ebook available soon

Library of Congress Control Number: 2020917531

Front cover photo by Ginger Ann Walker, back cover photo by Eddie Arnold, Sr,
Design by Nancy Arnold

For requests and inquiries, email the publisher: gingerwalker96@gmail.com

Visit my website
www.covid-19inreal-time.com

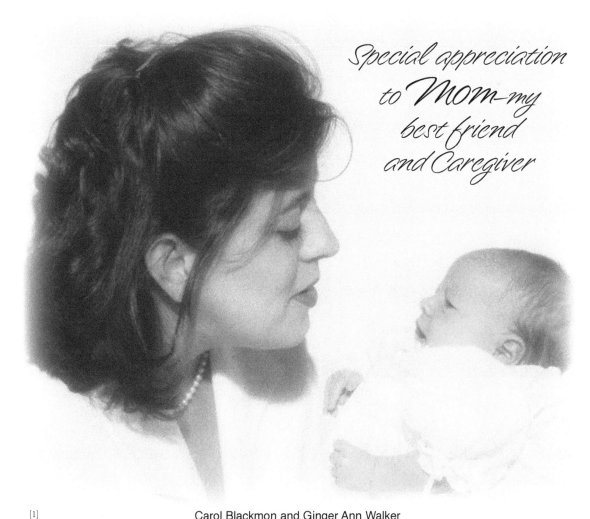

Special appreciation to Mom—my best friend and Caregiver

[1] Carol Blackmon and Ginger Ann Walker

M is for the many things [you] gave me,
O means only that [you are older].
T is for the tears [you] shed to save me,
H is for [your] heart of purest gold.
E is for [your] eyes with love-light shining,
R means right and right; [you'll] always be.
  —Put them all together; they spell **MOTHER**,
   a word that means all the world to me.

Adapted from *Mother* 1915—by Howard Johnson and Theodore Morse

Mom,

Abraham Lincoln first took my line when he said, "All that I am, or hope to be, I owe to my angel mother,"[1] Yet, he was only nine years old when she died. Considering the magnitude of her son's accomplishments, indeed, she had to be an incredible mother but no more so than mine!

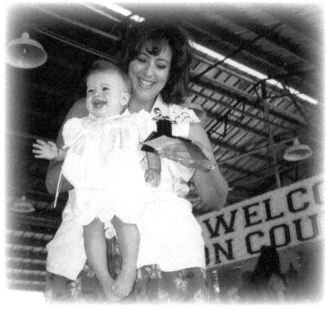

Ginger and her Mom, Carol, after winning the Blue Ribbon in [2] the Baby Pagent at the Wilson County Fair, 1997.

I read an anonymous quote stating that a person's real character, integrity, and strength cannot be measured until tested by adversity. Martin Luther King reinforced that notion when he said, "the ultimate measure of [a person] is not where they stand in moments of comfort and convenience, but in times of challenge and controversy."[2]

You have shielded me so often from adversities that this book would require a chapter to list them. This quality was especially evident at the lowest point of my life when the horrifying telephone call chilled me to the bone. I was too young and inexperienced to handle such shocking news, but when I turned to you, my rock, you were calm and steady as always. Without a word, your confident smile and tender touch assured me again you would be by my side no matter what I was about to face. Your strength had protected me for years from that imaginary killer whale, so indeed, by God's grace and your unwavering love, I became unafraid. I love you!

Ginger

INTRODUCTION

My Discovery of COVID-19

As a carefree child, I had little thought of the distant future; the world was my playground, and everything therein was good except for a killer whale I saw on television. I routinely asked at my bedtime tuck-in if he might get me in my dreams. It only was a child's fantasy, but I shudder to imagine how terrified I would have been from an actual glimpse into the future to see what was waiting to confront me 23 years later.

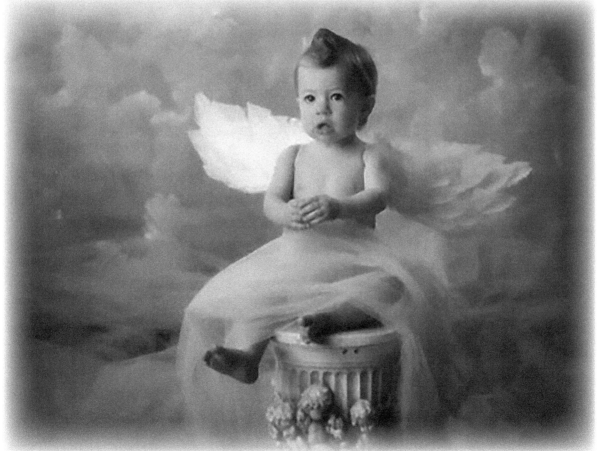

[3]

Ginger Ann Walker at 1 year old

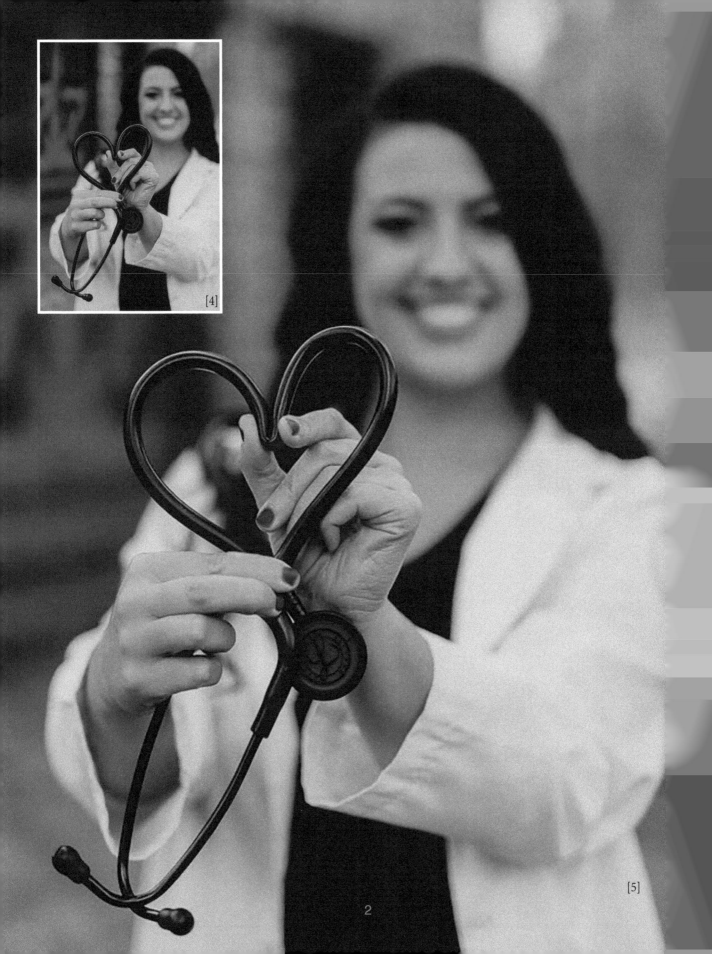

[4]

[5]

Observing patients with Covid-19 is worth a thousand words but is nothing like experiencing the disease in real-time

Writers Lee Thomas Miller, James Otto, and Jamey Johnson combined to pen Jamey's hit, "In Color."[3] It was one of my Grandad's all-time favorite songs partly because he was born in 1935, a featured line in the lyrics, and because he is such a big fan of Jamey's voice and music.

The clever lyrics compare hearing about challenges and tough times with the reality of experiencing them.

When employed as a nurse intern, I first met patients having symptoms of COVID-19. However, when I was diagnosed on June 5, 2020, as having the virus, I became an expert witness to its reality and implications. Initially, only the physical symptoms were available to prepare me for what to expect; however, I discovered there were formidable emotional and mental health challenges for which I had no warning.

Now that I have recovered. I feel an obligation to fill in the blanks. I offer to research scientists, doctors, nurses, patients, students, family members, and the general public, first-person information and support from my daily experiences. I dedicate my efforts to those who are infected, may become infected, are attempting to avoid infection, or are serving those who are infected. My story begins in early 2020 as a nursing school student at South College in Nashville. I also was employed as a nurse intern by Ascension Saint Thomas Midtown Hospital in Nashville, Tennessee.

I now have completed the final stages of my isolation from contracting COVID-19 and have received a serology test, indicating I have developed antibodies to SARS-CoV-2, the virus that causes COVID-19.

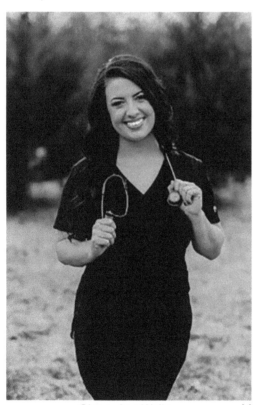
Ginger Ann Walker   [6]

According to the U.S. Food and Drug Administration (FDA), it is currently unknown if the presence of antibodies means I am immune to the virus in the future.[4] However, from all indicators, I am fully recovered, back at work, and feeling great.

Thank God for the special gift and opportunity to donate my blood containing antibodies to research and the treatment of seriously ill patients, battling for their lives.

TABLE OF CONTENTS

June 2020

SUNDAY	MONDAY	TUESDAY	WEDNESDAY	THURSDAY	FRIDAY	SATURDAY
31	Jun 1	2	3	4	5	6
7	8	9	10	11	12	13
14	15	16	17	18	19	20
21	22	23	24	25	26	2
28	29	30	Jul 1	2	3	

My Real-Time DAILY ACCOUNTS

					9	10
19	20	21	22	23	24	17
26	27	28	29	30	31	
2	3	4	5	6	7	[8]

6

DAY ONE, June 5, 2020. I woke up feeling great and looking forward to reporting to my work-station at Saint Thomas Midtown Hospital in Nashville, Tennessee, by 10:30 a.m. I left home early and stopped at a local drive-in for breakfast, which I hoped would sustain me for the long day—a 12-hour shift in the Emergency Department. I arrived ahead of schedule, and just before I entered to clock-in, I started feeling chest tightness on the right side. I suspected it was anxiety, or maybe I had eaten too hurriedly.

We especially were swamped on this particular day, such that it became necessary for me to administer at least 30 electrocardiograms. An ECG is an electronic test applied to detect heart problems and to monitor heart health.

A few hours into the shift, I became somewhat uneasy because my chest continued to feel abnormally tight. I asked one of the nurses to administer an ECG on me and found the results normal, so I continued working.

About halfway through my shift at 6:30 p.m., I felt extremely exhausted and tired, more so than in previous circumstances. I took my temperature, and because of a reading of 99.6°F—slightly high—the in-charge nurse arriving on duty sent me home. After I checked out, I informed my manager, who told me I would need to be tested for the Coronavirus before returning to work.

I went directly home and lay down to a night of deep sleep. Usually, I am never as tired after working only 6.5 hours!

DAY TWO, June 6, 2020. I woke up with additional symptoms. My lower back was hurting, and I had an excruciating headache behind my eyes. However, my chest tightness was not as severe as yesterday, and my temperature was only slightly elevated at 99°.

My symptoms had worsened—fatigue, fever, and other body aches. I knew my "work family" would take good care of me, so I checked into the Emergency Department as a patient around 1:00 p.m. and found my vital signs to be normal—blood pressure 120/80, heart rate 101 beats per minute, oxygen saturation 100%, and temperature 98.7°.

The doctor wanted to determine the state of my heart and lungs' by ordering an ultrasound, chest x-ray, and the COVID-19 test. I had administered it many times, but it was my first time to receive it. It involves inserting a six-inch-long swab into the nasal cavity. It is not unbearable but unpleasant enough to remind me to be more careful and empathetic with my patients in the future.

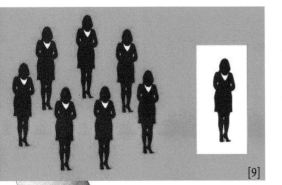
[9]

I had to wait quietly in a negative pressure room used for "airborne precautions," due to the suspicion that I am contagious. I wondered when my results would be reported, why it took so long, and what the future might hold.

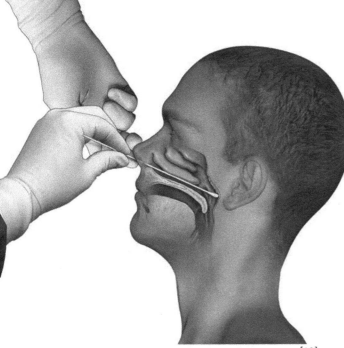
Courtesy of Medtronic.com [10]

The nurse completed the nasal swab. The X-ray tech came shortly to take the images, and while waiting for my results, I started reflecting on my time working in the E.R. (Emergency Room.) I usually take care of the patients, but now I am the patient and can better relate to their situation. When I return to work, I intend to be more considerate and patient with those challenged by fear, uncertainty, and worry. I once walked in their shoes.

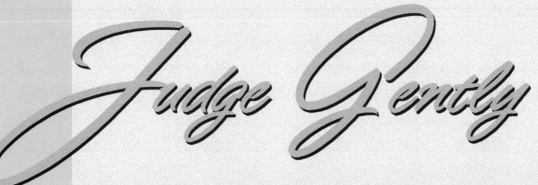

Judge Gently

Pray don't find fault with the man who limps

    or stumbles along the road,

unless you have worn the shoes, he wears

    or struggled beneath his load.

There may be tacks in his shoes that hurt,

    though hidden away from view,

or the burden he bears, placed on your back

    might cause you to stumble too.

Don't sneer at the man who's down today

    unless you have felt the blow

that caused his fall or felt the shame

    that only the fallen know.

— author unknown

Shortly, the doctor returned and concluded that I had right-sided pneumonia. The recommended treatment was taking the antibiotic, doxycycline—typically prescribed for pneumonia—for seven days. In fairness and complete objectivity, it was unknown at that time that it would be only a few hours before I would be diagnosed with the coronavirus, COVID-19. We ultimately learned that antibiotics such as doxycycline are ineffective on viruses.

However, we did not know if, in the early stages of treatment, doxycycline provided some mitigating benefits that expedited my recovery. I will leave that analysis to the doctors and scientists.

Nevertheless, the nurse discharged me and said they would call me when the nasal swab results arrived. I came straight home to lie down because the body aches were worsening, and I felt like two knives were stabbing me behind my eyes; It was quite severe. At about 9:00 p.m., a chilling phone call came to inform me that I had tested positive for Covid-19.

I had experienced adrenaline rushes a few times in my life as emotional responses to suddenly being frightened or scared—heart racing, palms sweating, and goosebumps. Still, that unnerving phone call stood the hair on the back of my neck like at military attention. I uttered a silent prayer of faith and trust; suddenly, a peaceful calm composed me, and my 14-day quarantine officially began. Fortunately, I escaped having to be placed on ventilation.

The basic regimen prescribed was to practice social distancing, wear a face mask in public, wash my hands frequently, not skip meals, take Tylenol for discomfort, and stay healthily nourished and hydrated. Remaining well-hydrated cannot be overly emphasized; I discovered it to be vital in my recovery process.

I am compliant with all the above, plus I now take a multivitamin and mineral supplement daily. At my own discretion, I added this after my research revealed that most patients admitted with COVID-19 are deficient in Vitamin D. Further, the zinc in my suppliment is receiving positive views from studies.

Practice Social Distancing	**Inside your home** *when someone has, or thinks they have, COVID-19. If possible, stay at least 6 feet away.* **Outside your home** *stay at least 6 feet away from people outside of your household in indoor outdoor spaces. Stay out of crowded places if possible.*

What is the difference between isolation, quarantine, and distancing?

Quarantine means restricting activities or separating people who are not ill themselves, but may have been exposed to COVID-19. The goal is to monitor symptoms and detect new cases early.	**Isolation** means separating infected people to prevent the spread of COVID-19.	**Physical distancing** means being physically apart but socially connected, for example through chat or video call.

[11]

As a people person, the constant separation from my family and friends was highly abnormal. I found it very frustrating and bewildering until I discovered that there is bliss hiding in solitude. I began my research into this malady that has taken over my life.

In isolation, recording my daily thoughts and experiences gave me a mission and purpose as a positive alternative to the maddening idleness. I determined that the appropriate starting point was to identify the enemy. I began with lots of reading, research, study, and documentation.

The World Health Organization is headquartered in Geneva, Switzerland, and was founded as a part of the United Nations after World War II. Its purpose is to alert the world to health threats and to fight diseases. There currrently are political issues and funding consequences over its neutrality and effectiveness, but that is another story for another day. My initial focus was on their role in reporting COVID-19 on January 21, 2020.

The following excerpt is taken from the first Coronavirus related World Health Organization Report: "On December 31, 2019, the World Health Organization China Country Office was informed of cases of pneumonia unknown etiology (unknown cause) detected in Wuhan City, Hubei Province of China. Within three days, through January 3, 2020, 44 case-patients with pneumonia of unknown etiology were reported.

"By January 20, 2020, only twenty days from the first report, the number had increased to 282 confirmed cases from four Asian countries. Twelve patients were in critical condition, and six had died.

"The World Health Organization, on February 11, 2020, named SARS-CoV-2 (severe acute respiratory syndrome) as the virus that caused COVID-19.[5]

"Within that initial month, on January 19, 2020, the first case in the U.S. was reported [subsequently disputed as being the first.] A 35-year-old man went to an urgent care clinic in Snohomish County, Washington, with a 4-day history of cough and subjective fever. After waiting for approximately 20 minutes, he was taken into an examination room and underwent an evaluation and the ultimate confirmation. He disclosed that he had returned to Washington State on January 15 after traveling to visit family in Wuhan, China.[6]

"Spreading like wildfire around 215 countries by July 26, 2020, there were 15,785,641 confirmed cases of COVID-19 and 640,016

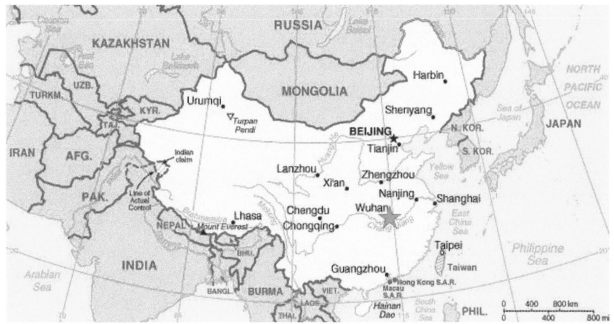

[12] The site of the original outbreak

confirmed deaths."

Wuhan is the most populated city in Central China, with over 11 million people. It is considered the nation's political, financial, and educational center.

Center for Disease Control and Prevention—The preceding original cause theory came from the U.S. Center for Disease Control, which described Covid-19 as a novel coronavirus—meaning that it previously had not been seen in humans. I learned that it is classified as zoonotic, meaning that it originated in animals and transferred to humans. For emphasis, the outbreak and the source were traced to the Huanan Seafood Wholesale Market, aka wet market, in Wuhan, China, in December 2019.

An alternative theory is that the virus was manufactured in a laboratory and released as a Chinese bioweapon. Twenty-seven prominent scientists from outside China disclaim this conspiracy notion. However, Dr. Li-Meng Yan, a Chinese virologist whistleblower, strongly disagrees. In September 2020, she claimed in several T.V. interviews to have evidence that the Chinese Government released the virus intentionally to create the pandemic.[7]

Although it is inconclusive if or which animals were part and parcel in hosting and transferring the virus, there is no dispute that the illness is transmitted primarily from person to person through respiratory droplets. Therefore, my initial focus was to research the potential connection animals might have had in my infection. After all, there are two dogs and three cats living in my home.

"I learned that 10 million dogs and 4 million cats are slaughtered for food each year, primarily in Asia. Their scientists and health specialists were concerned that the massive consumption of these animals pro-

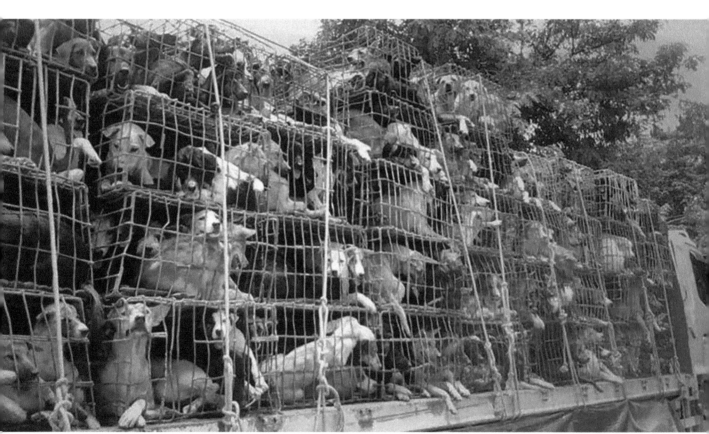

Dogs transported to the Wet Market [13]

cessed through their questionable wet markets placed them at high risk for infectious diseases.

"On May 1, 2020, Shenzhen, China, became the first city to legally ban eating cats and dogs. Recently Zhuhai, China, made a similar decision."[8]

These precautionary moves in China tended to justify my apprehension about the source of the infection. It is comforting for pet lovers that the Humane Society International consistently has upheld the principle that dogs and cats are companions and not for eating!

My research revealed there were more plausible carriers of the virus than family pets. According to the scienific community's original theory, horseshoe bats passed the virus to pangolin anteaters on to humans. The earlier belief that snakes were the missing link is disputed in favor of pangolins.

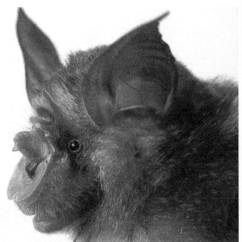 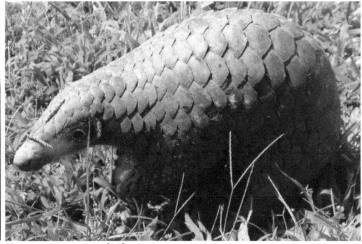

Horseshoe Bat [14]   Pangolin Anteater [15]

Accordingly, on September 13, 2007, The U.S. National Library of Medicine issued the following statement: "Horseshoe-nosed bats of several species… from different locations in the Southern People's Republic of China and the Hong Kong Special Administrative Region were found infected with SARS-like CoVs, and some of the bats had antibodies to these newly recognized viruses."[9]

Summary of the Early Stages

For the first time, on December 31, 2019, the world was informed about a mysterious unnamed virus in Wuhan City, Hubei Province of China. Approximately seven months later, on July 26, 2020, there were 15,785,641(including me) confirmed cases of the virus and 640,016 confirmed deaths. In nine months, COVID 19 has escalated from an outbreak to an epidemic (spread within a community, population, or region) to a pandemic (spread over multiple countries or continents.) The current statistics cite more than 30 million infected, and nearly one million to have died.

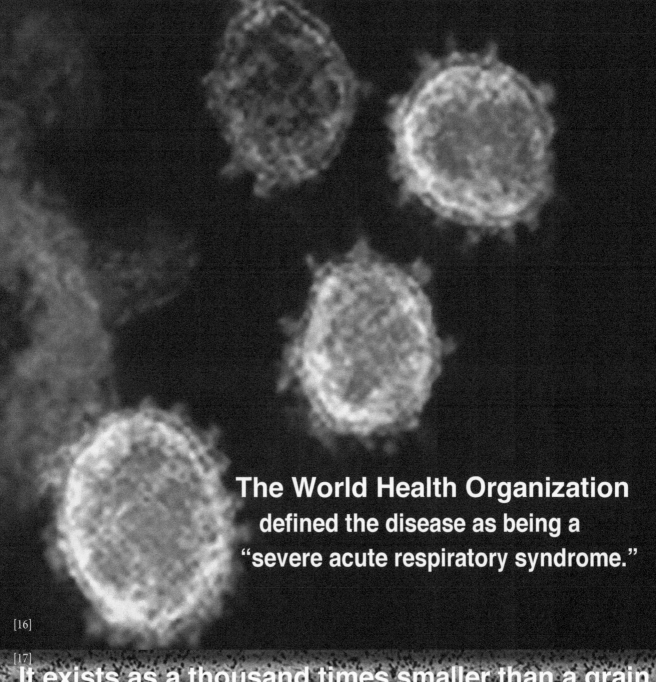

The World Health Organization
defined the disease as being a
"severe acute respiratory syndrome."

[16]

[17]
It exists as a thousand times smaller than a grain
of sand, and its primary function is to replicate.

Once infected, definitive symptoms will follow

The U.S. Centers for Disease Control offer the following symptoms, which may appear 2-14 days after exposure to the virus:[10]

- body aches
- chills
- congestion
- cough
- diarrhea
- difficulty breathing
- fatigue
- fever
- headaches

- loss of smell
- loss of taste
- muscle aches
- nausea
- runny nose
- shortness of breath
- sore throat
- vomiting

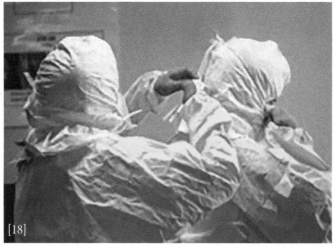

[18]

Nurses in protective clothing

The CDC offers the online Coronavirus Self-Checker link below to help individuals decide when to seek testing and appropriate medical care. If a reader has any of these life-threatening symptoms, please go to this website for the self-checker: help:https://www.cdc.gov/coronavirus/2019-ncov/symptoms-testing/coronavirus-self-checker.html

A skin turgor test for dehydration is appropriate as follows: Pinch the skin on the back of the hand and abdomen; if it does not snap back quickly, it indicates one likely is dehydrated.

Hydration Liquids St. Andrews University in Scotland tested and ranked common beverages for their impact on hydration.

Here's what they found, ranked from most hydrating to the least over four-hours. [11]

1. Skim milk
2. IV drinks*
3. Full-fat milk
4. Orange juice
5. Cola
6. Diet Cola
7. Cold tea
8. Hot tea
9. Sports drinks
10. Still water
11. Sparkling water
12. Lager
13. Coffee

* Electrolyte-enriched

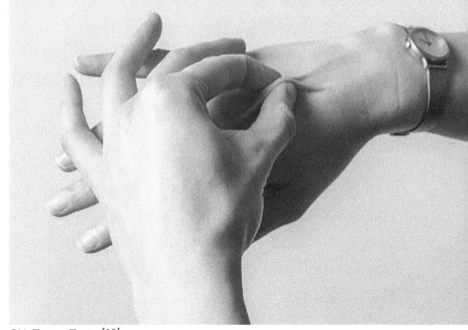

SkinTurgor Test [19]

The earlier conversations about my need to remain well-hydrated expanded my research to include all liquids, including energy drinks, a multi-billion dollar industry. Due to their popularity and attendant high levels of caffeine and sugar, an enormous health issue has emerged. "According to the Mayo Clinic, a typical 8-ounce cup of coffee contains around 90 mg of caffeine, about the same as a 2-ounce energy drink shot."[11a]

"Caffeine is relatively safe in small doses, such as in a cup of coffee or tea, but can be dangerous in amounts over 400 mg, according to an info sheet published by the University of California, Davis."[11b]

The consumption of multiple cups, cans, or bottles daily are common and easily exceed the 400 mg recommended limit. There are over 800 caffeinated energy drinks referenced on the internet. Several of them in the 8-ounce size contain over 300 mg of caffeine and up to 21 teaspoons of sugar. The American Heart Association limits healthy sugar consumption to 9 teaspoons full a day for men and 6 for women. Is it shocking to consider 21 teaspoons of sugar in a single energy drink?

Linking back ten years, "the Substance Abuse and Mental Health Services Administration (SAMHSA) reported more than 20,000 emergency room visits in the United States in 2011 involved energy drinks (doubled since 2007). More than half of those visits were due to energy drinks alone. The other cases involved people mixing alcohol or other stimulants with energy drinks."[12]

"According to the Center for Science in Public Interest, energy drinks were linked to 34 deaths since 2004." 2020 figures are unavailable but believed to be significant.

The excess intake of caffeine and sugar can cause: breathing issues, convulsions, diabetes, diarrhea, fatty liver disease, fever, heart attacks, high blood pressure, inflammation, irregular heartbeat, strokes, and weight gain.

"Energy drinks can be appealing to children and teens because they are available at local stores and are legal for all ages. According to the Centers for Disease Control and Prevention Trusted Source, 50 percent of teens say they consume energy drinks, and 75 percent of school districts do not have a policy regulating their sale on campus. In general, the regulation of energy drinks in the United States is lax. However, there is a movement calling for stricter regulation and content labeling and the addition of health warnings."

"Children and teens are particularly vulnerable to energy drinks as their bodies generally aren't used to caffeine. In one study, Trusted Source found that caffeine intoxication, or drinking too much caffeine, leads to caffeine addiction and potential withdrawal issues. The study concludes that energy drinks may be a gateway to other forms of drug dependence." [12a]

The daily limits of 400 mg of caffeine and 9 for men/6 for women teaspoons of sugar seem to be the consensus opinion; however, I hasten to defer to the medical professionals to advise their patients on caffeine and sugar matters. As a nurse, I have drawn my conclusions.

The National Academies of Sciences, Engineering, and Medicine guidelines for fluid intake from all sources are 15.5 cups (3.7 liters) for men and 11.5 cups (2.7 liters) for women. For emphasis, remaining hydrated is especially important for those recovering from COVID-19, and for general overall health benefits to everyone.[13]

The distinction used for describing weights merits further explanation for all readers. Most countries worldwide use the metric system for measuring the mass or weight of an object in grams. The prefixes kilo (1,000), milli (1/1,000), and centi (1/100) designate the magnitude. However, the United States continues to use the imperial system we inherited from the British at the time of colonization. It is helpful to understand both.

As a healthcare professional, I was required to learn how to convert units of measurement to the metric system. It is used throughout the medical profession because of its simplicity and its accuracy in administering medicine. The system is of French origin and is decimalized. Its magnitude changes by the power of ten by moving the decimal point to the left or right.

There often is confusion between mass or weight and volume when comparing ounces to liters. For example, soda is sold in liters, but milk and other liquids are sold by the gallon—a formula for confusion.

A standard plastic water bottle contains exactly 16.9 ounces in imperial measurement—an odd number of ounces but for a reason. It converts evenly to 0.5 of a liter, 500 milliliters, or a half liter in the metric system. One 2 liter soft drink bottle is equal to four 16.9 ounce bottles of any liquid.

Britain, the mother country of the imperial system, switched to metric in 1965. Still, the U. S., Myanmar, and Liberia remain the only three major countries to have retained the imperial system.[14]

Nevertheless, speaking within the United States' primary context and outside the medical circles in everyday lingo, I intend to drink the recommended eight (8 ounce) glasses or four (16.9 ounce) bottles of water every day.

DAY THREE, June 7, 2020. I woke up with a severe headache and lower back pain. Also, I am very weak and can barely walk to the bathroom without feeling exhausted. My temperature has stabilized at around 99°. I recently took a 1,000 mg Tylenol tablet for pain and drank a bottle of Biolyte,[15] a hydration drink recommended to address my somewhat dehydrated condition. Within a few minutes, I felt remarkably revitalized to the extent I wondered if it was the Tylenol or the hydration drink that perked me up so quickly. I never had been a user of electrolyte sports drinks, so I spent some time curiously researching this one's ingredients.

As a nurse, I am quite familiar with administering intravenous (IV) drip solutions at the bedside, generally to rehydrate or provide nutrients and medication to patients. Taking a so-called IV fluid orally was a new experience for me. I learned the one that I drank contained as many electrolytes as an IV bag or seven combined sports drinks. A doctor scientifically formulated it with chloride, sodium, potassium, and numerous vitamins. The Tylenol had alleviated my headache and back pain, but the invigorating feeling of well-being unquestionably came from the IV elixir, which at least temporarily was miraculous.

After several hours, the medication and fluids' effects began to dissipate, and I regressed somewhat. I returned to the Tylenol and Biolyte routine every eight hours, which made me feel better again and seemed to stabilize my condition.

Thankfully, I still have my smell, taste, and a good appetite. Also, my chest discomfort has improved. I only feel tightness and shortness of breath or experience coughing when I take a slow deep breath.

Since I was feeling somewhat better near the end of the day, it was a special treat to take a short, slow walk outside with my dog, who incidentally has not shown signs of abnormality. It was my first trip out of my house or bedroom, other than bathroom visits, and to get the meals left at my door. The fresh air, sunshine, and wooded trail were pleasant and refreshing. In accord with the Centers for Disease Control protocol, I wore a mask but did not come within sight of another person.

DAY FOUR, June 8, 2020. After such a refreshing day-ending walk yesterday, I am not off to a good start this morning; it is my worst so far. As the saying goes, perhaps it is the calm before the storm. I woke up in tears, tossing and turning with a nearly unbearable headache.

It took 1,000 mg Tylenol to hold it in check. However, my temperature was within the normal range at 99.5 degrees, and I still have a good appetite.

At mid-morning, I received a call from the Tennessee Department of Health, wanting to confirm my positive test results, which I have known for two days. The caller asked several general questions, including personal demographics, medical history, the development and evolution of the virus from my earliest symptoms, my home environment, and contacts up to three days before the onset of the virus. Then, she shifted to a wide variety of questions related to my boyfriend and his quarantine status.

She mentioned that he needed to quarantine himself for ten days longer than I, the one who exposed him to the virus. Nevertheless, he shows no symptoms and has had a negative nasal swab at this time. There is a chance he could be a carrier, and the virus "incubation period" is thought to be 10-14 days, although no one knows for sure at this time. Since I tested positive and developed symptoms, I am not at risk for "passively" infecting others, so I can come out of quarantine after ten days if I am absent from symptoms plus free of the medication regimen for at least 72 hours.

However, my employer's policy requires me to have two negative nasal swabs 24 hours apart before returning to work. At the end of the conversation with the lady from TDH, she assured me that someone from their department would be calling every day to follow up on how I am progressing.

My testimony as a nurse's perspective and from direct experience is that headaches are frequent and are horrendous for COVID-19 patients. Accordingly, by the afternoon, my headache was so intense, I decided to switch to an Aleve tablet. After 30 minutes, I almost was completely relieved. I call this reaction to the attention of research

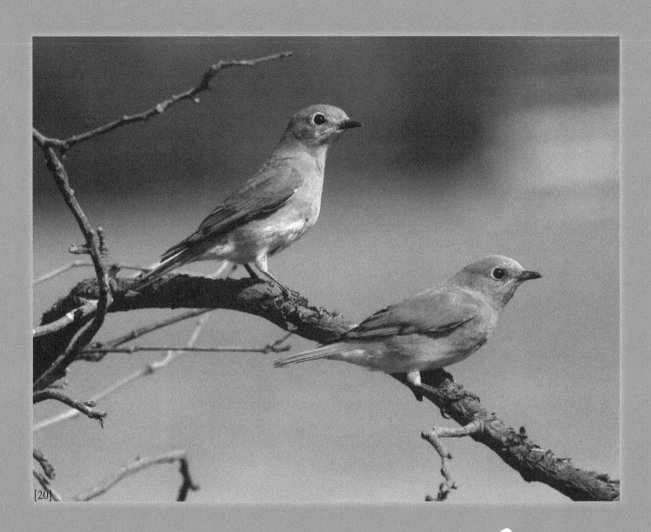

[20]

Social Distancing

scientists, doctors, and other health professionals. In this instance, a 220 mg tablet of Aleve (naproxen) was profoundly more effective than a 1,000 mg tablet of Tylenol (acetaminophen). It makes me wonder if COVID-19 symptoms respond better to the NSAIDs (Aleve and aspirin) than analgesics (Tylenol and generic acetaminophen). They are two different drug classes, but it was Aleve that enabled me to get out of bed and enjoy creating a piece of macramé wall art out of yarn. The relief and activity lifted my spirits and gave me hope that I had reached the illness's peak since I felt so much better. However, I had to remain cautious because I had taken Aleve previously without such a dramatic positive response.

I think it will be interesting to see what evidence is found related to these two drugs in the next few years. At this point, I was hopeful I had hit the peak of the illness since I felt so much better. My body was still weak and exhausted, but my pain was now at 2/10; progress!

DAYS FIVE, SIX, SEVEN, June 9,10, and 11, 2020. On day five, a very different symptom emerged—a progressive loss of smell and taste. It started when I was eating chocolate ice cream; it was cold and mushy, but no flavor. I knew that was a COVID-19 symptom, but it was an anomaly, unlike anything I had ever experienced.

By the end of day seven, a pattern had emerged. The daily symptoms continued with throat tickling, coughing, lack of smell and taste, leg cramps, tongue numbness, chest tightness, shortness of breath, and diarrhea. Strangely, I was quite hungry, although the thought of eating was repulsive.

The muscular pain became less frequent, but when needed, Aleve and Tylenol generally provided adequate relief. By day ten, my headaches had ended. Healthy balanced meals, a multivitamin and mineral supplement, the Biolyte hydration drink, along with frequent hand washing, and daily walks in my woods were standard inclusions in my daily regimen and routine.

Calls, cards, and flowers from friends and well-wishers were frequent, comforting, and appreciated.

I spent ninety percent of my time within four walls except for the short walks with my dog.

We are experiencing a rainy pattern lately— somewhat gloomy, but when the sun drives the clouds away, it is a special treat to be outside and to absorb some natural vitamin D. I am thinking positively, but there still is no joy inside solitary confinement.

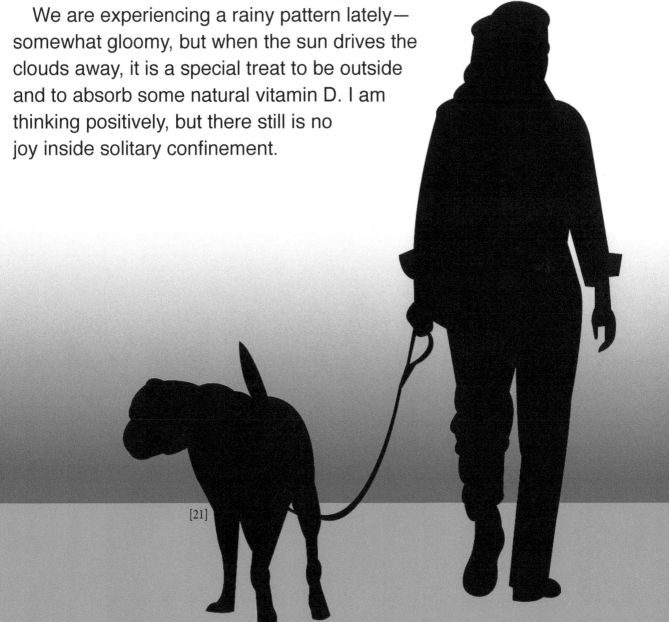

[21]

"I CAN SEE

[22]

CLEARLY
NOW
THE RAIN
IS GONE"

I Can See Clearly Now by Jimmy Cliff

DAY EIGHT, June 12, 2020. The pattern continues almost like a carbon copy of the first week. Certain peculiarities stand out, such as eating my favorite subway; it is like chewing on tasteless and odorless cardboard. The same goes for any other food, drink, or product. For example, I cannot smell shampoo when showering or the toothpaste when brushing my teeth.

This phenomenon is noticeable because the connection between the nose and mouth is through the same air passage, enabling smell and taste simultaneously. The adjustments to the physical handicaps require minimal effort and discipline. Still, the emotional and mental aspects, are crushing my spirit, and the recovery process is projected to last an additional six weeks. I stare at my room clock that appears frozen in slow-motion. My treatment regimen remains unchanged with Aleve and Tylenol for muscular pain and headaches, Biolyte for hydration, eating healthily, and regularly getting 8-10 hours of sleep.

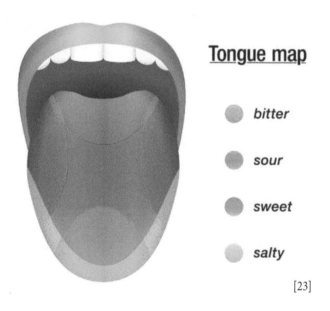

Tongue map

- bitter
- sour
- sweet
- salty

[23]

However, it is depressing and frightening, continually reading and hearing despair and doom statements such as this from Mayo Clinic doctors. "Currently, no medication is recommended to treat COVID-19, and no cure is available. Antibiotics aren't effective against viral infections such as COVID-19. Researchers are testing a variety of possible treatments. Clinical trials seeking a cure continue rapidly around the world, but with minimal success. Dexamethasone has been shown to reduce deaths in patients requiring mechanical ventilation and oxygen. There are claims of success using

Hydroxychloroquine and Azithromycin. However, the U. S. Food and Drug Administration and the World Health Organization have stopped hydroxychloroquine testing because the results were not encouraging and, in some instances, proved to be harmful."[16a]

I am not half-way through my quarantine period, yet the idleness in this isolated environment is continuing to wear on me. The anguish extends beyond what television can relieve or satisfy. I must immediately develop coping mechanisms that challenge the confinement that is haunting and depressing me. I emphasize with all my zeal and urgency the importance of filling every waking moment with "things to do" that are constructive and time-consuming in a positive sense. I am open to suggestions.

When I first gave thought to write a book about my journey to, thru, and from COVID-19, I dismissed the notion because I felt clueless about the entire process. I had no training, experience, or confidence to do it, although I thought my message could help the scientific community, doctors, patients, and the general public.

Perhaps it was providential that my Dad and Granddad had completed the Dale Carnegie course years ago. It is designed to help build greater self-confidence, strengthen people skills, enhance communication skills, develop leadership skills, and control worry and stress. *How to Win Friends and Influence People* is the program's flagship self-help book written by Dale Carnegie and published in 1936.[17] Over 30 million copies have been sold worldwide, making it one of the best-selling books of all time. In 2011, it was number 19 on Time Magazine's list of the 100 most influential books.

My Granddad gave me a copy a couple of years ago, which I read with interest, but the component focusing on worry and stress renewed my attention. Soon, I was talking to a former Carnegie instructor who opened my eyes with thought-provoking revelations. I shared my feelings of inadequacy, and his response was so inspiring that I can almost quote it word for word.

"Ginger, you are the world's greatest authority speaking and writing about yourself and your experiences. No one can tell your story better, so simply relate it as your memory recalls. Even if you forget and leave out something, no one will know the difference because they did not experience it in the first place."

His encouragement was compelling enough to reassure me and strengthen my confidence, but there was more. After I told him I planned to focus on the stress-related issues that were my most significant emotional and mental obstacles, he raised an unusual question.

He asked if I ever had read the story of *Alice in Wonderland?* [18]

I had not, so he proceeded
to tell me all about it.

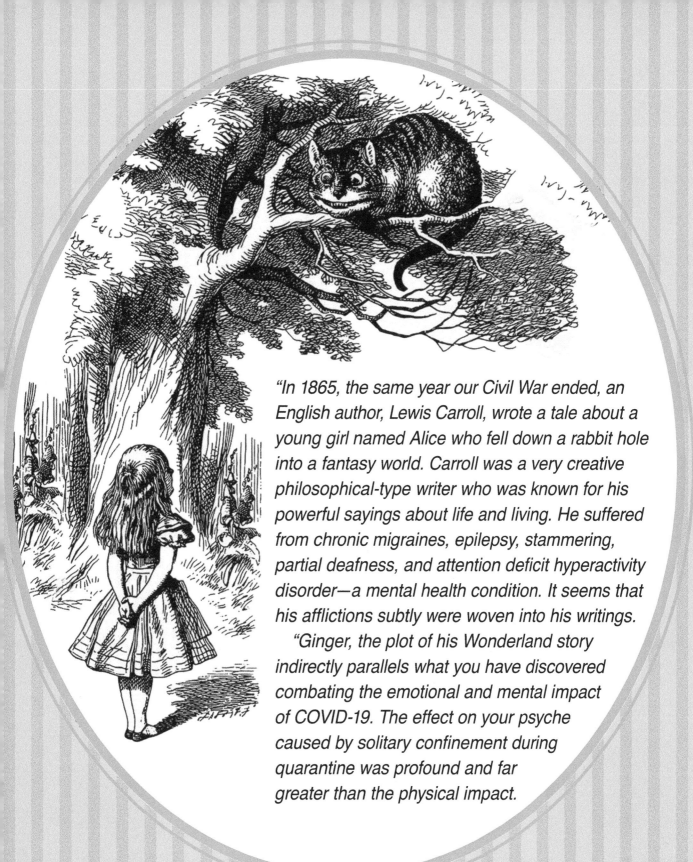

"In 1865, the same year our Civil War ended, an English author, Lewis Carroll, wrote a tale about a young girl named Alice who fell down a rabbit hole into a fantasy world. Carroll was a very creative philosophical-type writer who was known for his powerful sayings about life and living. He suffered from chronic migraines, epilepsy, stammering, partial deafness, and attention deficit hyperactivity disorder—a mental health condition. It seems that his afflictions subtly were woven into his writings.

"Ginger, the plot of his Wonderland story indirectly parallels what you have discovered combating the emotional and mental impact of COVID-19. The effect on your psyche caused by solitary confinement during quarantine was profound and far greater than the physical impact.

"In Carroll's make-believe Wonderland, there were countless objects and animals isolated from the real world. They could talk and were personified with human characteristics, emotions, and behaviors; foremost, all had mental illnesses, perhaps developed from being secluded from unaffected people and normalcy.

"Health care professional Maria Giulia Marini determined that Alice suffered from hallucinations and personality disorders; the White Rabbit from General Anxiety Disorder; the Cheshire Cat with Schizophrenia, as he disappears and reappears distorting reality around him; the Queen of Hearts was affected by egotism and Narcissist syndrome, the hookah-smoking Caterpillar by drug addiction, and the Mad Hatter, simply by madness.

"Even a neuropsychological condition was adopted as the story's name, i.e., Alice in Wonderland Syndrome (AIWS), also known as Todd's Syndrome or Dysmetropsia. It is a condition that distorts perception. The distortion may occur for other senses besides vision. Indeed, it seems the Wonderland resembled a type of asylum for the mentally ill."[18a]

"Throughout Carroll's life and writing career, he was preoccupied with the subject of mental illness and the incarceration of patients. His uncle, Skeffington Lutwidge, was a Commissioner for inspecting so-called lunatic asylums. Many of his uncle's colleagues in psychiatry also became his friends.

"Consider the strange dialog between Alice and the Cheshire Cat who told her that everyone isolated in the rabbit hole was 'mad'; not mad in a temperamental sense, but 'mad' as being seriously mentally ill.

So Ginger, in a sense, you and all COVID-19 patients who find yourselves restricted to living in solitary confinement, are indeed in a potentially maddening environment. "A United Nations reporter, Juan Mendez, and widespread numbers of mental health reformers assert that isolation of more than 15 days could amount to torture. Scientific studies have established that lasting mental damage can be caused after only a few days of social isolation."[18b]

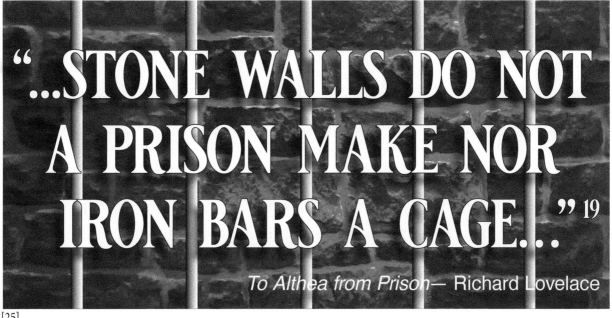

"...STONE WALLS DO NOT A PRISON MAKE NOR IRON BARS A CAGE...."[19]

To Althea from Prison— Richard Lovelace

[25]

I was curious throughout my discussions with the Carnegie instructor about how he was so in touch with mental illnesses due to aloneness, incarceration, and isolation-by choice or unavoidable circumstances. Upon questioning, I learned he had served in the Navy as a hospital corpsman and a neuropsychiatric technician. He had assisted doctors and other medical professionals in the care and treatment of patients who had developed profound emotional and mental disorders. In many instances, they were dangerous to themselves and others. Consequently, he mostly was attuned to how the brain and the rest of the nervous system influences a person's cognition and behaviors.

He described my antagonist in military hospital terms as psychological torture, more commonly known as "White Torture." It was standard procedure decades ago to lock-up patients if they were thought to be faking illnesses to escape strict discipline and the extreme regimentation. It involved isolating the prisoners in separate all-white soundproof cells designed to suppress all of their senses. They were prohibited from talking to anyone, nor hearing anything except for themselves. Many adverse effects result from this form of torture. It forces the detainee to lose personal identity and can even cause hallucinations. Prisoners often are kept in these rooms for months or even years.

The instructor described the horrors of solitary confinement as cruel and inhumane treatment similar in many respects to the archaic practice of bloodletting. The procedures usually did not improve the disorders and typically made them worse.

My new friend's opinion that the recent upsurge in alcohol and substance abuse, suicides, domestic violence, psychiatric disorders, and an array of other general health issues is stress-related, resulting from the extraordinary numbers of people being quarantined. It is far worse now than in the 2007-2009 recession when the suicide rates in the United States and Europe claimed over 10,000 lives.

Leo Sher reinforces the forgoing in his writing for the QJM Journal of Medicine: "the psychiatric effects of the COVID-19 crisis will become progressively evident in the coming months and years as the consequences of chronic anxiety, prolonged distress, physical distancing, loneliness, death of friends and family members and employment losses manifest. It is vital to take proactive steps to minimize the detrimental impact of the coronavirus pandemic on mental health."[20]

The Carnegie instructor's motive was to influence me to identify stress-relieving activities that will address the numerous illnesses plaguing those secluded in solitary confinement.

One of the main characters which Alice met in the Wonderland was a Cheshire cat. He has been immortalized for decades in the simile, "grinning like a Cheshire Cat."

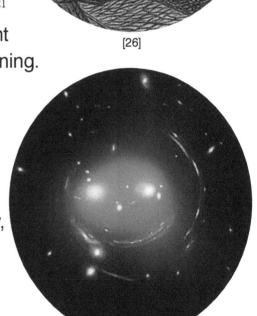

A further snippet indirectly related is that The National Aeronautics and Space Administration (NASA), Albert Einstein, and the Cheshire Cat shared a common relationship.[21]

Einstein's unusually high Intelligent Quotient compared to the average of 98 merits mentioning. According to the best measurements available at that time, his IQ was 160, which is in the 99.998 percentile of all test takers.[22] His brilliance led him to devise his theory of special relativity ($e=mc^2$), which revolutionized our understanding of space, time, and gravity, and led to the Atomic Bomb's creation. A related coincidence for me is that one of the last living developers of components for the bomb, Mary Boswell, lives across the street from where my Mom grew up.

As the cat suggested to Alice in the Wonderland narrative, my writing leads me down interesting trails I did not initially plan to go; I am amazed. According to NASA, Alice in Wonderland was the inspiration behind the name given to a group of Galaxies. The Chandra X-Ray Observatory released the image above in 2015 and nicknamed the group the Cheshire Cat galaxies. Some of the "cat" features are distant galaxies, whose light has been stretched and bent by gravitational lensing.

While Alice was searching to find her way out of that stressful underground environment, she came to a fork in a road and found the

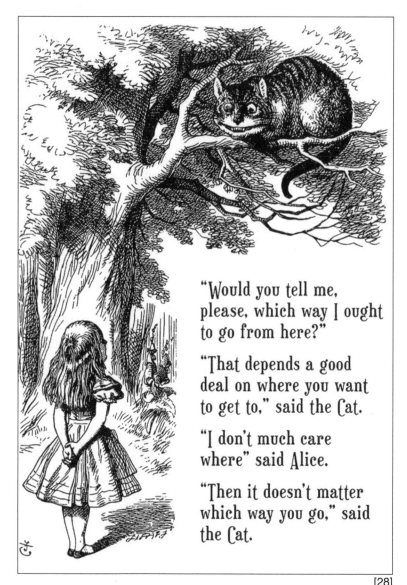

"Would you tell me, please, which way I ought to go from here?"

"That depends a good deal on where you want to get to," said the Cat.

"I don't much care where" said Alice.

"Then it doesn't matter which way you go," said the Cat.

[28]

omnipresent Cheshire Cat perched in a tree. Alice asked him which road she should take? The cat asked her where she wanted to go, and Alice said she did not know. The wise cat then advised her that if she didn't know where she wanted to go, any road would take her there —good advice for all life decisions.

"So Ginger, there is a parallel to the Cheshire Cat's common sense advice and conclusions. Since you are an authority on the plot of the book you wish to write, sit down and start writing, and your thoughts will complete it for you. It will take you down a trail for which you could not plan before the fact. The twists, turns, hills, valleys, and detours will wait for you en route. In other words, you are not sure in general terms where your narrative will take you until you get there.

"Time management is an important first step to help you reduce long-term stress by giving you direction when you work from a plan and schedule. It puts you in control of where you are going and helps you to increase your productivity."

He shared that stress, anxiety, and depression can cause forgetfulness, confusion, difficulty concentrating, and other abnormal problems that can disrupt one's life. In profound cases of amnesia, he related that, in his experience, the patients were locked in padded jail-like cells and in straightjackets to restrain them from physically harming themselves.

His message seemed so straight forward yet life-changing. I am uncertain where this project is taking me, but I expect to arrive at a destination in due time. The risks to me and other recovering COVID-19 patients dealing with intense stress, anxiety, and depression, have captured my utmost attention.

As we concluded our conversation, the instructor emphasized sufficient direct and implied evidence that Carroll portrayed what can happen to people in prolonged isolation and confinement. He had more to tell me in another session we planned in the coming days.

The Dale Carnegie course is a viable option for patients quarantined more so than ever since it now can be taken online. My Grandad is a big fan of the program as evidenced by his declaration that he found it more beneficial to his career than his six years of college.

Warren Buffett, the seventh richest man in the world, joins the other famous business tycoons in this image of his bookcover crediting the value of the Dale Carnegie program to their success.

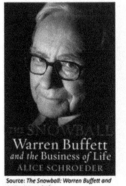

"My Dale Carnegie certificate is the most important degree I have."

a. Emeril Legasse
b. Mary Kay Ash
c. Warren Buffett
d. Bill Gates
e. Sam Walton [Wal-Mart Founder]

Warren Buffett
and the Business of Life
ALICE SCHROEDER

Source: The Snowball: Warren Buffett and the Business of Life

[29]

It now is **DAY NINE**, June 13, 2020, only eight days into my quarantine segment of this continuum leading to parts unknown. In his *House by the Side of the Road*, Sam Walter Foss creatively phrased how I view my journey.

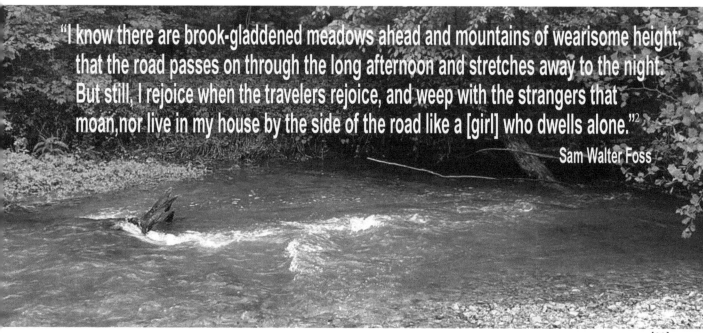

"I know there are brook-gladdened meadows ahead and mountains of wearisome height; that the road passes on through the long afternoon and stretches away to the night. But still, I rejoice when the travelers rejoice, and weep with the strangers that moan, nor live in my house by the side of the road like a [girl] who dwells alone."[2]

Sam Walter Foss

[30]

If my healing progresses well, it will be July before I am released to return to my job. I have been free of headaches for three days, which I believe is a major turning point.

It is apparent that a pattern is established. The aches and pains are not as frequent, and when they do occur, Aleve and Tylenol provide significant relief. Healthy balanced meals, a multivitamin and mineral supplement, the Biolyte hydration drink, along with daily walks, continue as my standard regimen and routine.

Physically, I feel I am continuing to improve; however, the nemesis remains entrenched—the emotional and mental pressures resulting from isolation are worsening. It is a morbid thought, but I have no assurance that I will get well and fulfill my dreams to nurse the sick and infirmed—my chosen career and "calling" for which I have spent years in preparing.

In the next session with the Carnegie instructor, I became convinced of the urgency that I immediately must address this destructive confinement. He observed that I am spinning my wheels in the process because I have not narrowed my focus to a plan of action. Accordingly, I was introduced to a strange-sounding analogy known as the "law of parsimony" or Occam's Razor.

William of Ockham

William was an English Franciscan friar, theologian, and philosopher (circa 1287–1347.) remembered primarily for a saying attributed to him and named for him as Occam's razor.[24] In basic terms, it is a problem-solving technique whereby multiple options are "shaved" away, leaving only the simplest solution. In other words, processes should not be multiplied without necessity. An answer to a problem or decision that requires the fewest assumptions is generally the best choice. Professor

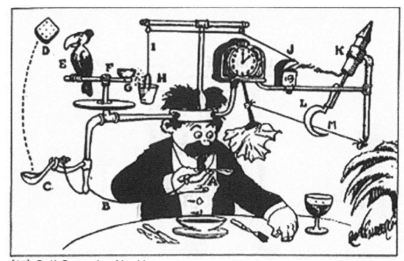

[31] Self-Operating Napkin

Butts demonstrates the iverse of the law.

"The soup spoon (A) is raised to the mouth, pulling string (B) and thereby jerking the ladle (C), which throws the cracker (D) past the toucan (E). The toucan jumps after the cracker and the perch (F) tilts, upsetting seeds (G) into the pail (H). The extra weight in pail pulls the cord (I), which opens and ignites the lighter (J), setting off skyrocket (K), which causes the sickle (L) to cut the string (M), allowing the pendulum with the attached napkin to swing back and forth, thereby wiping his chin."

"Ginger, Rube Goldberg, the creator of this illustration was a turn of the century cartoonist and the only person ever to be listed in Merriam-Webster's Dictionary as an adjective.[25] You will notice in his napkin invention, he multiplied the processes unnecessarily. He made the simple task of wiping one's mouth with a napkin, as Occam's Razor would suggest, into a complex mechanism with multiple variables.

"I will involve you in a parallel example for further emphasis. Let's say you came home from work and found trash scattered all over the floor near a tipped over trash can. There are several possible explanations for what has happened:

    a. A burglar broke into your home and sorted through the trash can looking for valuables.

    b. Your dog knocked the can over to get a morsel of food.

    c. The fan on the central air system sped up due to an electrical malfunction increasing the suction through the vents to such a force it turned over the trash can.

As you can conclude, (a) and (c) have multiple assumptions, but (b) has reduced the number of unsupported assumptions in the explanation; therefore, you reduced the likelihood of being wrong if you choose b.

"Ginger, I cannot overemphasize Occam's Razor as a tool to help you determine which activities you should include in your 'things to combat stress' list. Occam's maxim of choosing the simplest of multiple choices is reinforced further by the famous scientist Isaac Newton, 'We are to admit no more causes of natural things than such as are both true and sufficient to explain their appearances. Therefore, to the same natural effects, we must assign the same causes as far as possible.'

"Perhaps a greater coincidence to the Wonderland analogy and your quandary is expressed in this Newton quotation, 'I can calculate the motion of heavenly bodies, but not the madness of people.'

"Most importantly, Ginger, tell me how you plan to choose the activities to occupy your idleness."

I responded that I planned to ask for the opinions of my family, friends, and professionals with specializations in areas of my interest. A benefit of being quarantined is my emergence to recognize and appreciate the amazingly diverse influences I have within my immediate family and friends. There is an accountant, administrator, athlete, artist, auctioneer, author, builder, coach, collector, entrepreneur, fisherman, hunter, investor, musician, salesman, seamstress, singer, stenographer, and teacher; along with cats which rub against my legs as they purr their affection, and dogs that wag their tails in approval of every expression of kindness.

Each seems to have a different role to model for me. As I observe them, I learn many important things about life and living that extend beyond material values. Amazingly, several are multitalented. They are knowledgeable and compitant in a number of fields. They wear many hats equally well.

"I am a part of all I have met."

Ulysses—Alfred Lord Tennyson

"All the world's a stage, and all the men and women merely players; they have their exits and their entrances; and one man in his time plays many parts...

As you like it—WIliam Shakespeare

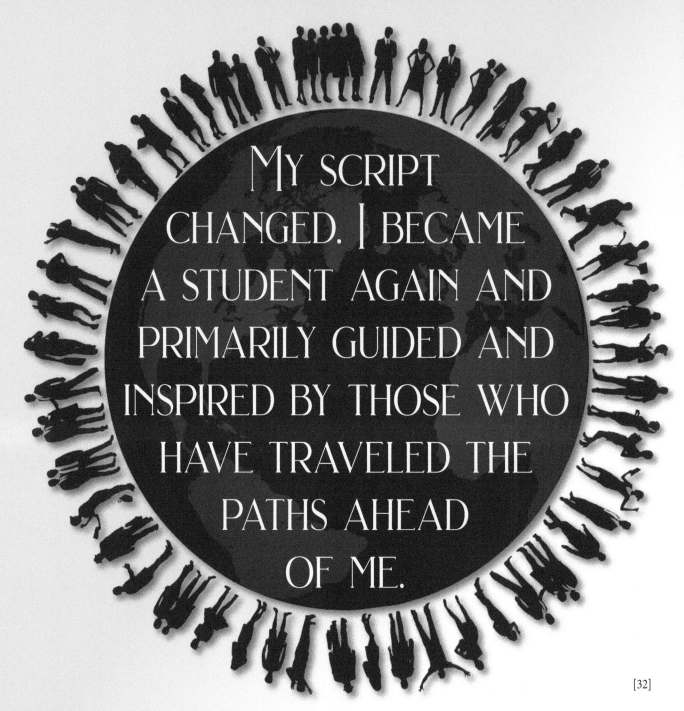

MY SCRIPT CHANGED. I BECAME A STUDENT AGAIN AND PRIMARILY GUIDED AND INSPIRED BY THOSE WHO HAVE TRAVELED THE PATHS AHEAD OF ME.

[32]

My paternal grandmother, Nanny Lu Walker, an expert seamstress, taught me several projects for my idle time within the sewing domain. The quilt image on pages 114 and 115 are of a "get well" gift she and Aunt Julie made and is evidence of her remarkable sewing skills. She designed and crafted incomparable children's' clothes that I cherished and proudly wore from my earliest memories.

More importantly, she consistently demonstrated and continues to project what my Dale Carnegie coach emphasized as the most admirable traits people should develop. Nanny Lu is the personification of Dale Carnegie's master list, starting with her wonderful disposition. I never have heard a negative word from her lips nor seen a scowl on her face. Collectively, her low-key manner, humility, and measured confidence project a magnetic personality that magically draws people to her. She has inspired me to study self-help books and tapes from which I can learn, practice, and polish what seems so natural for her. During my research, I found numerous examples that reinforce the importance of "personality" in influencing my relationship with people and my career. I came upon a comical example to illustrate:

A particular couple in a local office consistently displayed disagreeable and offensive dispositions—birds of a feather. No matter the situation, a gloomy "rain on the parade" expression would transform a beautiful day into one of doom and gloom. The predicate of their every response included what likely could go wrong. It was so depressing even to be in their negative presence was avoided by other workers.

One morning, the couple arrived with a pleasant smile on their faces, which prompted an observer at break time to mention the change in their usual negative manner. He asked in wonderment what on earth had happened to them; why did they seem so happy? A quick-witted responder remarked, "they must have heard some bad news."

A highly achieving executive, life coach, and author, Shawn Doyle, reinforces the notion that most successful people make it a rule to avoid associating with complainers, grumps, and poor-mouthers. Toxic individuals with destructive attitudes, especially those who believe the world has jinxed them, tend to get in our heads, poison our thinking, and drain our productive energy.

Joe Btfsplk, Al Capp's hard-luck character from Lil'l Abner comics, brought disaster and misfortune to himself and everyone around him

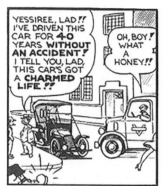
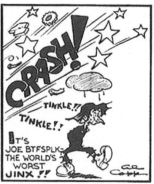

[33]

as a dark cloud hung over him everywhere he went. His luck was so bad he is believed to be the only person in the world without a vowel in his name.

Conversely, a positive thinker, Carlisle Beasley, shared with me a compelling parallel found in the word "attitude." Its numerical position in the alphabet is the only word in the dictionary that cumulatively adds up to 100%. Attitude has everything to do with one's countenance, disposition, manner, nature, outlook, optimism, self-control, and temperament.

Audible.com offers a remedy to those desiring personality improvement in the form of 30 days of free listening to *How to Win Friends and Influence People.*

A	1
T	20
T	20
I	9
T	20
U	21
D	4
E	5
	=100%

[34]

THE OPTIMIST (From several versions)

I passed a sandlot yesterday, and some kids were playing ball.
I strolled along the third-base line within the fielder's call.
"Say, what's the score?" I asked the chap, and he yelled to beat the stuffin'
"There's no one out, the bases are full, and
    they're forty-two to nuthin!"
"You're getting beat, aren't you, my lad?"
And then in no time flat, he answered,
"No sir, not as yet! Our side ain't been to bat!"

—*Tumblin Creek Tales* by Richard M. "Pek" Gunn

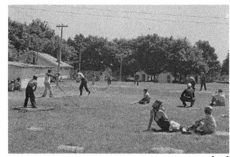

[35]

Thank you, Nanny Lu, for sharing your good attitude with me. I plan to follow your example.

My parents and grandparents on both sides, especially, have been guiding lights for me. Their varying talents and shared life experiences have been positive influences. So, I began my query with them, seeking their suggestions on ways and means of becoming and remaining productive within my quarantined environment.

My Maternal Grandmother, Nannie, received my first inquiry. She is remarkably youthful in looks and spirit for one who is past eighty-four. Her life experiences and accomplishments are incredible examples of how determination can overcome meager resources and challenging circumstances.

She is very reluctant to boast because she believes those who do usually are offensive to others, and beneath their bluster, often an inferiority complex is exposed. They are not great enough to be humble. Accordingly, she suggested that I perform my work in a manner worthy of praise, but not to seek it; and to ignore the critics. She offered lines from President Teddy Roosevelt's *Man in the Arena* to reinforce her advice:

> *"It is not the critic who counts; not the man who points out how the strong man stumbles, or where the doer of deeds could have done them better. The credit belongs to the man who is actually in the arena, whose face is marred by dust and sweat and blood; who strives valiantly; who errs, who comes short again and again, because there is no effort without error and shortcoming; but who does actually strive to do the deeds; who knows great enthusiasms, the great devotions; who spends himself in a worthy cause; who at best knows, in the end, the triumph of high achievement, and who at the worst, if he fails, at least fails while daring greatly, so that his place shall never be with those cold and timid souls who neither know victory nor defeat."* [26]

Regardless, I cannot resist tooting her horn a bit as evidence of the kind of credible resources I am seeking to counsel me. I want guidance from exceptionally successful people, not the ordinary. Her modesty will cause her to cringe and wince upon reading that I publically shared her resume.

In high school, college, and work career, she was a high achiever athletically, academically, and pro-fessionally. Her superlatives include being all-state in basketball, achiev-ing straight A's in high school and

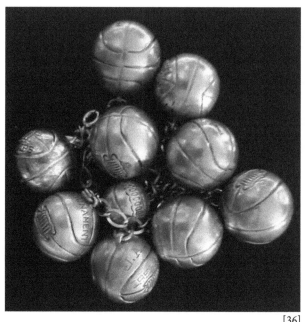

[36]

My grandmother's all-star and most-valuable awards in the 1950's

college, to become the youngest person ever to be an Administrative Assistant to the Chief Justice of the Supreme Court of Tennessee, and one of only two peers to earn the nations highest stenographical award—National Certified Professional Secretary.

In this role on the state's highest court, she regularly interfaced with the most notable public servants, legal minds, and brilliant thinkers in Tennessee and Washington, D.C. Therefore, with high confidence in her frame of reference and informed judgment, I asked her what she thinks is the best application of my many hours of free time during my quarantine. "Become broadly informed by reading widely and working crossword puzzles" was her simple reply! Nannie is prolific in the daily practice of both.

Reinforcing her recommendation is Nikita Bhagat,[27] author at wealthordsworth.com says, "Crossword puzzles are more than just a pastime activity. Being a boredom buster, they are actually beneficial to our mental and physical health." [Beyond the basic entertainment] The additional benefits include:

1. Improved Vocabulary
2. Lessened Stress
3. Increased Social Bonding
4. Improved Mental Health
5. Improved Cognitive Functioning
6. Increased General Knowledge."

The availability of Crossword puzzles, along with jigsaw puzzles and countless word games, usually is common knowledge starting with the daily newspapers, magazines, and internet links.

"idle hands are the devil's workshop: idle lips are his mouthpiece Proverbs 16:27-29

After some thought, Nannie suggested that I expand my resource base by seeking opinions from a cross-section of people in my network via telephone or text since I cannot expose them to possible infection. I should ask them to share their ideas about cultivating useful activities to become involved while being isolated. I am anxiously waiting to be cleared to report to the first day of my career as a professional nurse. Meanwhile, I am frustrated and bored nearly out of my mind.

Nannie's parting advice was to frame every decision made in my life's journey and the current project on my acceptance and trust in God, the Supreme Being—Omnipotent, Omnipresent, and Omniscient; and treating all people as I wish to be treated. Accordingly, the Nightingale Pledge embodies my committment:

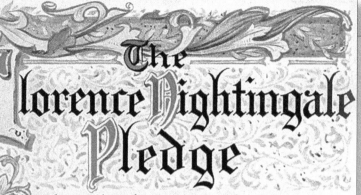

I solemnly pledge myself before God and in the presence of this assembly, to pass my life in purity and to practice my profession faithfully. I will obstain from whatever is deleterious and mischievous, and will not take or knowingly administer any harmful drug. I will do all in my power to maintain and elevate the standard of my professing, and will hold in confidence all personal matters committed to my keeping and all family affairs coming to my knowledge in the paractice of my calling. With loyalty will I endevor to aid the physician in his work, and devote myself to the welfare of those committed to my care.

The Founder of Modern Nursing

Within the constraints of my lockdown, I indeed became closer to God. It is not as a so-called deathbed conversion—a religious change of heart when one faces the potential of the end of life. I have been grounded in my faith since early childhood at home and church. As well, my assignment in the Emergency Room of a major hospital indirectly places me in touch with that fleeting moment daily. From my viewpoint, I never have met an atheist among those medical professionals who regularly witness the miracle of life suspended in its most fragile circumstance. COVID-19 is transformative in many ways, including one's spiritual perspective.

Following Nannie's advice, I immediately began building my repertoire of idle time activities. Books and puzzles were my first two entries.

I was introduced to several bookworms known as bibliophiles because of their love for books and the multiple benefits reading provides. My great-uncle Bill, in particular, was a prolific reader. Perhaps he was motivated in part because of his profound hearing loss. In a sense, he was quarantined somewhat the same as we with COVID 19.

He traveled widely but lightly with one change of clothes and at least four books in his handbag. He was a walking encyclopedia, a whiz with crossword puzzles, and possessed a massive vocabulary likely enhanced because of his advanced literacy level. He was recognized as the outstanding city manager of the year in the United States. His brother, my Granddad, believed his role was enhanced primarily as a result of his depth of knowledge and skills gained by being an intense reader.

Granddad has a copy of his brother's list from which he read his entire life. I have included it for my use and others who may find it helpful:

Bill's Recommended Reading List

A. All-time best-selling books of more than 100 million each.
   a. The *Bible* - multiple authors   5 billion
   b. *The Quran* - Muhammed   800 million
   c. *The Tale of Two Cities* - Dickens   200 million
   d. *The Little Prince-de Saint* - Exupéry   150 million
   e. *Harry Potter* - Rowling   120 million
   f. *The Hobbit* - Tolkien   150 million
   g. *Then There Were None* - Christie   100 million
   h. Dream of the Red Chamber-Cao Xueqin   100 million
B. *The Harvard Classics* - An anthology compiled and edited by Dr. Charles W. Eliot, Harvard University president in 1909. Dr. Eliot is credited with saying that the elements of a liberal education can be obtained by reading only 15 minutes a day from these classics.
C. The *Great Books of the Western World*, a 54 volume set published in 1952. Robert Hutchins collaborated with Mortimer Adler to develop a course to render the reader as an intellectually rounded man or woman familiar and knowledgeable of the great ideas developed in the course of three thousand years.
D. http://read.gov/books/ This web address links to hundreds of free online classic books for all ages at the Library of Congress.

An October 2019 *Healthline* article cited research showing that regular reading improves brain connectivity, increases vocabulary and comprehension, empowers empathy with other people, aids in sleep readiness, reduces stress, lowers blood pressure and heart rate, fights depression symptoms, prevents cognitive decline as one ages, and contributes to a longer life.[28]

The Well Educated Mind

Susan Bauer suggests in her book "The Well-Educated Mind, a Guide to Classical Education You Never Had,"[29] an excellent list of great books from five genres as below:

Fiction:

1. *Don Quixote* - Miguel De Cervantes
2. *The Pilgrim's Progress* -John Bunyan
3. *Gulliver's Travels* - Jonathan Swift
4. *Pride and Prejudice* - Jane Austen
5. *Oliver Twist* - Charles Dickens
6. *Jane Eyre* - Charlotte Bronte
7. *The Scarlet Letter* - Nathaniel Hawthorne
8. *Moby Dick* - Herman Melville
9. *Uncle Tom's Cabin* - Harriet Beecher Stowe
10. *Madame Bovary* - Gustave Flaubert
11. *Crime and Punishment* - Fyodor Dostoyevsky
12. *Anna Karenina* - Leo Tolstoy
13. *The Return of the Native* - Thomas Hardy
14. *The Portrait of a Lady* - Henry James
15. *Huckleberry Finn* - Mark Twain
16. *The Red Badge of Courage* - Stephen Crane
17. *Heart of Darkness* - Joseph Conrad
18. *The House of Mirth* - Edith Wharton
19. *The Great Gatsby* - F. Scott Fitzgerald
20. *Mrs. Dalloway* - Virginia Wolfe
21. *The Trial* - Franz Kafka
22. *Native Son* - Richard Wright
23. *The Stranger* - Albert Camus
24. *1984* - George Orwell
25. *Invisible Man* - Ralph Ellison
26. *Seize the Day* - Saul Bellow
27. *One Hundred Years of Solitude* - Gabriel Garcia Marquez
28. *If on a Winter's Night a Traveler* - Italo Calvino
29. *Song of Solomon* - Toni Morrison
30. *White Noise* - Don DeLillo
31. *Possession* - A.S. Byatt
32. *The Road* - Cormac McCarthy

Autobiography:

1. Augustine - *The Confessions*
2. Margery Kempe - *The Book of Margery Kempe*
3. Michel De Montaigne - *Essays*
4. Teresa Of Avila - *The Life of Saint Teresa of Avila by Herself*
5. Rene Descartes - *Meditations*
6. John Bunyan - *Grace Abounding in the Chief of Sinners*
7. Mary Rowlandson - *The Narrative of the Captivity and Restoration*
8. Jean Jacques Rousseau - *Confessions*
9. Benjamin Franklin - *The Autobiography of Benjamin Franklin*
10. Frederick Douglass - *Life and Times of Frederick Douglas*
11. Henry David Thoreau - *Walden*
12. Harriet Jacobs - *Incidents in the Life of a Slave Girl, Written by Herself*
13. Booker T. Washington - *Up from Slavery*
14. Friedrich Nietzsche - *Ecce Homo*
15. Adolf Hitler - *Mein Kampf*
16. Mohandas Gandhi - *An Autobiography: Story of Experiments with Truth*
17. Gertrude Stein - *Autobiography of Alice B. Toklas*
18. Thomas Merton - *Seven Storey Mountain*
19. C.S. Lewis - *Surprised by Joy: the Shape of my Early Life*
20. Malcolm X - *The Autobiography of Malcolm X*
21. Maya Angelou - *I Know Why the Caged Bird Sings*
22. May Sarton - *Journal of a Solitude*
23. Aleskandr Solzhenitsyn - *The Gulag Archipelago*
24. Charles W. Colson - *Born Again*
25. Richard Rodriguez - *Hunger of Memory: Education of Richard Rodriguez*
26. Jill Ker Conway - *The Road from Coorain*
27. Elie Wiesel - *All Rivers Run to the Sea*

History/Politics

1. Herodotus - *The Histories*
2. Thucydides - *The Peloponnesian War*
3. Plato - *The Republic*
4. Plutarch - *Lives*
5. Augustine - *The City of God*
6. Bede - *The Ecclesiastical History of the English People*
7. Niccolo Machiavelli - *The Prince*
8. Sir Thomas More - *Utopia*
9. John Locke - *The True End of Civil Government*
10. David Hume - *The History of England, Volume V*
11. Jean-Jacques Rousseau - *The Social Contract*
12. Thomas Paine - *Common Sense*
13. Edward Gibbon - *The History of the Decline and Fall of the Roman Empire*
14. Mary Wollstonecraft - *A Vindication of the Rights of Woman*
15. Alexis De Tocqueville - *Democracy in America*
16. Karl Marx and Friedrich Engels - *Communist Manifesto*
17. Jacob Burckhardt - *Civilization of the Renaissance in Italy*
18. W.E.B. Du Bois - *The Souls of Black Folk*
19. Max Weber - *The Protestant Ethic and Spirit of Capitalism*
20. Lytton Strachey - *Queen Victoria*
21. George Orwell - *The Road to Wigan Pier*
22. Perry Miller - *The New England Mind*
23. John Kenneth Galbraith - *The Great Crash*
24. Cornelius Ryan - *The Longest Day*
25. Betty Friedan - *The Feminine Mystique*
26. Eugene D. Genovese - *Roll, Jordan, Roll: The World the Slaves Made*
27. Barbara Tuchman - *A Distant Mirror: The Calamitous Fourteenth Century*
28. Bob Woodward and Carl Bernstein - *All the President's Men*
29. James McPherson - *Battle Cry of Freedom: The Civil War Era*
30. Laurel Thatcher Ulrich - *A Midwife's Tale: The Life of Martha Ballard*
31. Francis Fukuyama - *End of History and the last Man*

Drama:

1. Aeschylus - *Agamemnon*
2. Sophocles - *Oedipus the King*
3. Euripides - *Medea*
4. Aristophanes - *The Birds*
5. Aristotle - Poetics
6. Everyman (14th Century)
7. Christopher Marlowe - *Doctor Faustus*
8. William Shakespeare - *Richard III*
9. William Shakespeare - *A Midsummer Night's Dream*
10. William Shakespeare - *Hamlet*
11. Moliere - *Tartuffe*
12. William Congreve - *The Way of the World*
13. Oliver Goldsmith - *She Stoops to Conquer*
14. Richard Brinsley Sheridan - *The School for Scandal*
15. Henrik Ibsen - *A Doll's House*
16. Oscar Wilde - *The Importance of Being Ernest*
17. Anton Chekhov - *The Cherry Orchard*
18. George Bernard Shaw - *Saint Joan*
19. T.S. Eliot - *Murder in the Cathedral*
20. Thornton Wilder - *Our Town*
21. Eugene O'Neill - *Long Day's Journey into Night*
22. Jean Paul Sartre - *No Exit*
23. Tennessee Williams - *A Streetcar Named Desire*
24. Arthur Miller - *Death of a Salesman*
25. Samuel Beckett - *Waiting for Godot*
26. Robert Bolt - *A Man for All Seasons*
27. Tom Stoppard - *Rosencrantz and Guildenstern are Dead*
28. Peter Shaffer - *Equus*

Poetry:

1. *The Epic of Gilgamesh*
2. Homer - *The Iliad and the Odyssey*
3. Greek Lyricists
4. Horace - *The Odes*
5. *Beowulf*
6. Dante Alighieri - *Inferno*
7. *Sir Gawain and the Green Knight*
8. Geoffrey Chaucer - *The Canterbury Tales*
9. *William Shakespeare - Sonnets*

10. John Donne
11. King James Bible - Psalms
12. John Milton - *Paradise Lost*
13. William Blake - *Songs of Innocence and of Experience*
14. Williams Wordsworth
15. Samuel Taylor Coleridge
16. John Keats
17. Henry Wadsworth Longfellow
18. Alfred, Lord Tennyson
19. Walt Whitman
20. Emily Dickinson
21. Christina Rossetti
22. Gerald Manley Hopkins
23. William Butler Yeats
24. Paul Laurence Dunbar
25. Robert Frost
26. Carl Sandburg
27. William Carlos Williams
28. Ezra Pound
29. T.S. Eliot
30. Langston Hughes
31. W.H. Auden

Science

1. Hippocrates - *On Airs, Waters and Places*
2. Aristotle - *Physics*
3. Lucretius - *On the Nature of Things*
4. Nicolaus Copernicus - *Commentariolus*
5. Francis Bacon - *Novum Organum*
6. Galileo Galilei - *Dialogue Concerning the Two Chief World Systems*
7. Robert Hooke - *Micrographia*
8. Isaac Newton - excerpts from *Philosophiae Naturalis Principia Mathematica*
9. Georges Cuvier - *Preliminary Discourse*
10. Charles Lyell - *Principles of Geology*
11. Charles Darwin - *On the Origin of Species*
12. Gregor Mendel - *Experiments in Plant Hybridization*
13. Alfred Wegener - *The Origin of Continents and Oceans*
14. Albert Einstein - *The General Theory of Relativity*

15. Max Planck - *The Origin and Development of the Quantum Theory*
16. Julian Huxley - *Evolution: The Modern Synthesis*
17. Erwin Schrodinger - *What is Life?*
18. Rachel Carson - *Silent Spring*
19. Desmond Morris - *The Naked Ape*
20. James D. Watson - *The Double Helix*
21. Richard Dawkins - *The Selfish Gene*
22. Steven Weinberg - *The First Three Minutes:*
23. A Modern View of the *Origin of the Universe*
24. E. O. Wilson - *On Human Nature*
25. James Lovelock - *Gaia*
26. Stephen Jay Gould - *The Mismeasure of Man*
27. James Gleick - *Chaos: Making a New Science*
28. Stephen Hawking - *A Brief History of Time*
29. Walter Alvarez - *T. Rex and the Crater of Doom*

Best Life Website

40 Books You Hated in High School That You'll Love Now - link to https://bestlifeonline.com/classic-books/

I regret to admit that I have read very few of the great classics and all-time favorite books. In fact, I am a slow reader and do not comprehend well. Frankly, I did not enjoy reading for pleasure until my Granddad told me about an amazing reading phenomenon from his high school days who rarely took books home to study. His school provided a daily "study hall" in their library where students could do research and "get their lessons." Every six-weeks their English teacher required students to complete reading a library book and give a summary report about it in front of the class.

The amazing part of Granddad's account is that Bobby would select his book from the library shelves only an hour before he was scheduled to deliver his report. As the story goes, Bobby would stand with confidence and poise in front of the class and summarize the book with the eloquence of an orator as though he had written it.

One day, Bobby shared his method as to how he was able to accomplish such a feat. He said that 15 minutes of concentrated study is worth more than 15 hours interrupted by distractions, diversions, and daydreaming. Secondly, he demonstrated he could "speed-read" a typical non-technical book in 30 minutes by scanning only the topic sentence of each paragraph (the main idea) and the entire paragraph (the summary) at the end of each chapter.

Also, he would sweep his index finger and skim read rapidly by skipping phrases and modifiers focusing on nouns and verbs. For example, "inside the storage room, the tall boy was able to reach up high to the top shelf and remove the shoebox for his much shorter teacher." He essentially would read the words highlighted in red and his brain would grasp the context and automatically fill in the blanks. Ironically, significant research indicates that increased reading speed improves comprehension.

Evelyn Wood, who founded a famous speed-reading course con-

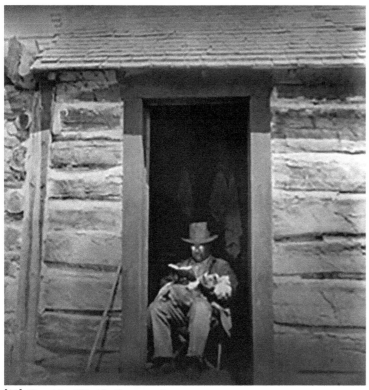
[38] President Teddy Roosevelt

firmed that reading faster actually increases retention. Staff members of three presidential administrations received her training. Mrs. Wood was timed with reading speeds of 6,000 words a minute and demonstrated her capability by reading a 689 page book with comprehension in less than an hour.[30]

President Theodore Roosevelt is reputed to have read one book every morning before breakfast and three books per day.

As a young man, President John F. Kennedy was a slow reader with a speed less than 300 words per minute. He increased his speed four times to 1,200 per minute by learning to read words in groups he referenced as "thought units."

Professional typists function similarly by typing letters and words in groups. For example, their brains think of the word "the" as one whole unit not as t-h-e. As their skill level improves, so does their eye and hand coordination, enabling them to type phrases of three or more words. My previously referenced grandmother won the business education award in high school typing over 100 words per minute without errors and on a manual typewriter.

The human mind works wonders with just a few context clues. The point of this is we tend to read too slowly and not enough.

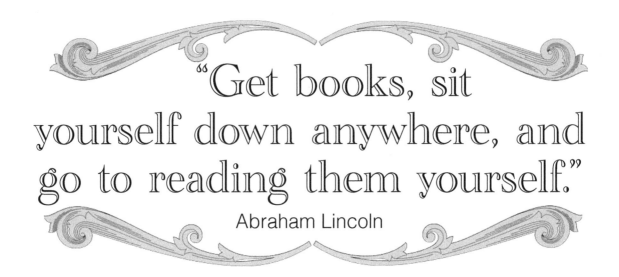

> "Get books, sit yourself down anywhere, and go to reading them yourself."
>
> Abraham Lincoln

A READER LIVES A THOUSAND LIVES BEFORE HE DIES, SAID JOJEN. THE MAN WHO NEVER READS LIVES ONLY ONE.[31]

George R. R. Martin

Fortunately I encountered another incredible resource person, a speed-reading specialist. Susan is a retired educator who formerly prepared college students for the enormous reading challenges as they transitioned from high school to college. She volunteered a week to help me improve my reading skills via Zoom, a cloud platform for video and audio conferencing, chat, and webinars. She has helped me double my reading speed in a week basically using the same technique used by Bobby in the foregoing account nearly 60 years ago.

I miraculously have been liberated by this new speed-reading skill and I am falling in love with the content of books. For practice, I shocked myself by reading a 200 page novel in one day!

I am pondering and reading more than ever, even trying my hand at creative writing as evidenced by this project. The power in words is more meaningful than ever before and the talent of authors and composers more appreciated. When I happen upon phrases that really strike me as worthy and relevant, I find a place in this narrative to share them with my readers.

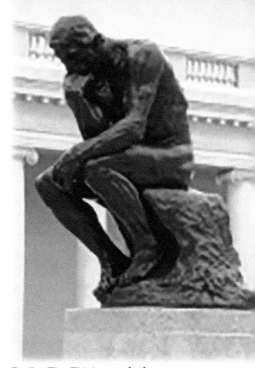

Rodin, The Thinker   [39]

My Granddad, as an educator, sharpened my focus on the elegance and influence contained within words and particularly those in the English language. In retirement, he taught English as a second language to refugees and immigrants.

He explained why English is extraordinary and magical, yet very difficult to learn as a second language. His reasoning is because of the countless words which are spelled the same and sound the same but have different meanings—homonyms. For example, the word "set" has 200 meanings, "run" has 645 meanings, and "take" has over 1000 meanings, all depending on the context in which the words are used; accordingly, there is a run of luck, a home run, a run in her hose, a run for the rabbits, a run for mayor, etc.

I especially find warmth and comfort in lines and lyrics in music such as in this popular tune from my grandparents' 50's era, "Little Things Mean a Lot." [32]

> Give me your hand when I've lost the way, Give me your shoulder to cry on, whether the day is bright or gray give me your heart to rely on . . .

The sometimes controversial but oft-quoted Yehuda Berg described the capability of words in a most captivating way, "Words are singularly the most powerful force available to humanity. We can use this force constructively with words of encouragement or destructively using words of despair. Words have energy and power with the ability to help, to heal, to hinder, to hurt, to harm, to humiliate, and to humble.[33] Yet, in truth, we rarely understand the influence our words have on others and especially on ourselves.

"Without words, our thoughts cannot become a reality. Words describe our mood, our opinions, and our emotions. They enable us to communicate with others and build relationships. And perhaps most importantly, we use words to describe to ourselves who we are and our future path. In this way, I believe words have their ultimate power in influencing a life of positivity or one of difficulty and despair."

DAY TEN, June 14, through **DAY TWENTY FOUR** on June 28, essentially was like a looping song in terms of my physical feelings. My daily regimen remained unchanged except for saturated reading persuits and adding new activities to my arsenal.

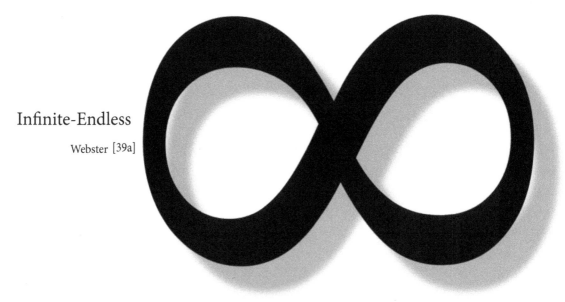

Infinite-Endless

Webster [39a]

The 21st was father's day and I reminded him of the old saying that a son is a son until he takes a wife, but your daughter is your girl for all of her life. We had a good conversation but still kept our social distance. My dad taught me the value of a strong work ethic and more importantly, demonstrated the characteristics as long as I can remember.

I woke up today, the 22nd with no fever, headache or pain! My nose is stopped up but my cough feels loose. Mom made blueberry pancakes. I ate all of them, but still without taste. Later, I had my blood drawn and was tested positive for antibodies. It is too early to be assured that I have immunity, so I must continue to practice social distancing and follow the CDC health regulations.

Back to the continuing curse—the torture of solitude. Increasing my reading activity has been a good diversion from twiddling my thumbs in idleness. Two weeks of phone interviewing with dozens of amazing achievers has been very productive. I have learned and added several incredible "things to do" to my bag of options. I am excited to share with others educational and cultivating activities that have elevated the quality of my quarantine and my life in general. Hopefully, they will be helpful to others with or without COVID-19.

Nothing has changed in my daily routine so it is a good point to introduce my new discoveries.

To Do List

1- read a book
2- take Knox for a walk
3- work crossword puzzle
4- read Dale Carnige
5- work on narrative
6-

[40]

Benefits of Memorization
—Poetry and Song Lyrics—

The best and most eloquent public speakers I have ever heard were in the pulpits of various churches; and were politicians delivering persuasive messages framed to influence voters. I cannot recall but few instances where lines of poetry or song lyrics were not used to reinforce their themes or specific points.

According to Tony Robbins, the famed motivational speaker, "the two greatest orators of antiquity are Cicero and Demosthenes. When Cicero was done speaking, people always gave him a standing ovation and cheered, 'What a great speech!' When Demosthenes was done, people said, 'Let us march,' and they did. That's the difference between presentation and persuasion." [34]

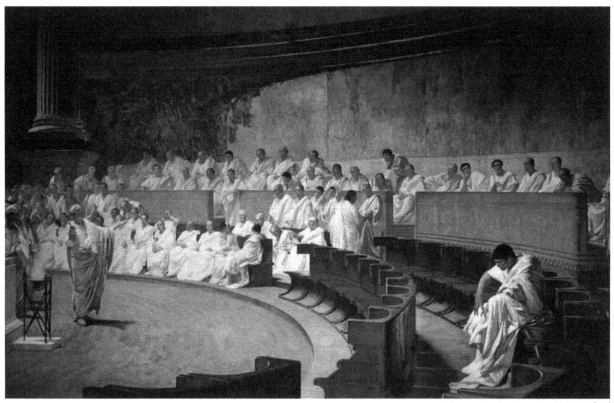

Cicero in the Roman Senate [41]

The classical poets memorized hundreds and even thousands of lines of their epic poems as a means of preserving them. In the absence of printing presses, the only other alternative to the tedious hand copying with quill pens was rote memory. For example, the Greeks were able to orally pass down Homer's Iliad and Odyssey despite there being nearly 28,000 total lines between them. Would that feat not use all of the brain's capacity to achieve it?

A well known myth exists that even the genius Albert Einstein only used 10% of his brain capacity. neurologist Barry Gordon at Johns Hopkins School of Medicine in Baltimore says that " we use virtually every part of the brain, and that [most of] the brain is active almost all the time."[35]

Regardless, IQ scores above 135 place a person in the 99th percentile, so Einstein's lofty 160 suggests that ordinary folks need not be concerned about depleting or over-filling their memory reservoir with extensive amounts of information.

A November 2010 article in Stanford Medicine News by Mark Tuschman revealed that "A typical healthy human brain contains about 200 billion nerve cells, or neurons, linked to one another via hundreds of trillions of tiny contacts called synapses.One synapse can store 4.7 bits of information."[36]

To place this immensity in perspective, my Grandmother, Nannie, as a highschool cheerleader recalled a "cheer" phrased as: "two bits, four bits, six bits, a dollar, all for Springfield, stand up and holler." Therefore, in a money conversion, one snapses equals about 59 cents and when multiplied by hundreds of trillions of synapses, the sum approaches an infinite number.

CNS (Clinical Neurology Specialists) neurologists along with numerous reputable sources further corroborate the enormity of the human brain's storage capability as trillions of bytes of information. [37]

I learned an interesting notion practiced by my Granddad as he did his walking exercise. He would commit a favorite poem or song lyric to memory by continuing his walk until the words were fixed in his mind. He termed it, "mental gymnastics" which eliminated the boredom of the activity while enhancing the health benefit.

Subsequently, he would apply perfectly matched memorized lines in his speeches, writings, and general conversation to reinforce a point or values lesson. He emphasized that memorization is a skill improved by habitual repetition (rote) and is one of the main principles in developing a command of language. It was used in the teachings of the ancient Greek philosophers, poets, historians, gifted writers, and orators.

I recall an example of this application that happened during a phone call inquiry late one stormy night. Our conversation was interrupted by tapping on the door of my quarantined room by Mother checking to see if I needed anything before she retired. Although I was feeling lousy, there was nothing she could do for me. Like turning on a light, Granddad quickly drew from his memory bank of hundreds a parallel and quoted:

> "Once upon a midnight dreary, while I pondered, weak and weary, over many a quaint and curious volume of forgotten lore— While I nodded, nearly napping, suddenly there came a tapping, as of someone gently rapping, rapping at my chamber door. Tis some visitor, I muttered, tapping at my chamber door—only this and nothing more." [38]

I instantly loved it and was smitten by the words that incredibly paralleled my situation and the moment. He said it was taken from the poem, *The Raven,* written by Edgar Allan Poe, who died prematurely at the age of 40, possibly from Cholera.

The diagnosis intrigued me because the symptoms of Cholera are similar to some of the signs of Covid-19, i.e., dehydration, fatigue, sunken eyes, a dry mouth, extreme thirst, and skin that is slow to bounce back when pinched. That kinship quickly was dismissed when I remembered that Cholera is caused by a bacterial infection whereas Covid-19 is from a virus.

Sadly, I learned that Poe sold the Raven for nine dollars, and it soon became a worldwide bestseller. In December 2009, a first-edition copy of one of his poem books sold at Christie's in New York City for $662,500.[39]

The value of this example illustrates how a simple poem or lyric occupied my mind, opened windows of knowledge, and entertained me for hours while exploring the many factual links launched by the words and life of this master poet. Perhaps it explains why I also have become fascinated and more attuned to powerful words and phrases found in other poems, prose, and song lyrics. I plan to borrow from them to enrich my writing throughout this narrative.

Accordingly, each day I am memorizing a verse or more of a poem and recommend the practice to all who are living in isolation for any reason. It is good for the mind and spirit.

Evan Mantyk, president and co-founder of the Society of Classical Poets, offers his opinion of the ten greatest poems ever written for our consideration.

All-time Greatest Poems [40]

1. *Sonnet 18* by William Shakespeare (1564-1616)
2. *Holy Sonnet 10: Death, Be Not Proud* by John Donne (1572-1631)
3. *Daffodils* by William Wordsworth (1770-1850)
4. *A Psalm of Life* by Henry Wadsworth Longfellow (1807-1882)
5. *On His Blindness* by John Milton (1608-1674)
6. *The Tiger* by William Blake (1757-1827)
7. *Ode on a Grecian Urn* by John Keats (1795-1821)
8. *Ozymandias* by Percy Bysshe Shelley (1792-1822)
9. *The New Colossus* by Emma Lazarus (1849-1887)
10. *The Road Not Taken* by Robert Frost (1874-1963)

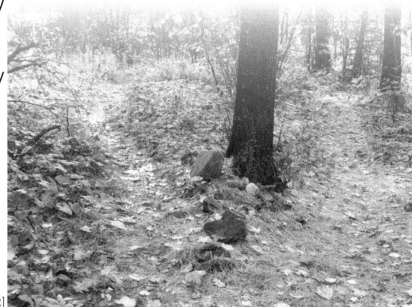
[42]

Dr. William R. Klemm writing in *Psychology Today* made a strong case for the importance of memorization to good mental health:[41]

> *"Memorized information is always with you, even when you lack the time or access to sources where you could look it up. We think and solve problems with what is in working memory, which in turn is the memory of currently available information or recall of previously memorized information.*
>
> *"The process of thinking is like streaming video on the Internet: information flows in as short frames onto the virtual scratchpad of working memory, successively replaced by new chunks of information from real-time or recalled memory. Numerous studies show that the amount of information you can hold in working memory is tightly correlated with IQ and problem-solving ability."*

Song Lyrics

To me, song lyrics and poetry are close to the same thing. Certainly there are technical differences such as with the melody that typically accompanies lyrics. However, the words and messages of both formats are inseparable in terms of their beauty and fulfillment. Classic song lyrics are no more nor less creative than classic poetry.

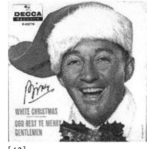
[43]

"May your days, be merry and bright…" In this best selling single of all time, Bing Crosby sang Irving Berlin's *White Christmas* and sold over 50 million copies. Michael Jackson's *Thriller* remains the best-selling album of all time, with sales of 66 million copies. Obvious the lyrics of favorite songs heard repeatedly are more quickly memorized and retained as poetry. Soon after learning to walk, my younger brother could recite hundreds of lines of Michael Jackson's hits.

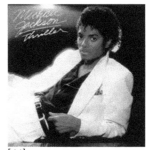
[44]

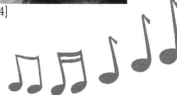

Music Therapy

According to an article in *Eurica Alert,* December 2014 issue, as early as 4000 BC, *hallelujah to the healer* was played as part payment for medicinal services, while the ancient Greeks identified Apollo as the father of both healing and music.[42]

More recently, studies have shown beneficial calming and even pain relieving effects of music for patients having surgery.[1]

As stated, I consider song lyrics nothing more or less than poems set to music. There are many parallels such as rhythm, theme, mood, meter, rhyme, stanza, and line.

---

1. https://www.sciencedaily.com/releases/2014/12/141211210036.htm

Similar to aerobics, listening to music reduces levels of the body's stress hormones—adrenaline and cortisol. It also stimulates the production of endorphins, the body's natural mood elevators. Ninety percent of surgeons listen to music during surgery, according to a survey conducted by Spotify.[43]

Catherine Meads, an author of a study at Brunel University in the United Kingdom, "found that patients who listened to music either before, during, or after surgery had less pain, took less pain medication and were less anxious after surgery. The effects lasted more than four hours.[44]

"The researchers also found that patients seemed to benefit no matter what type of music they heard."

The following is an excellent link to history's top music for
Lyric Memorization Practice:
https://en.wikipedia.org/wiki/List_of_best-selling_singles

In summary, memorizing lines in poems and lyrics in songs enhances the neurological flexibility of the brain. "University researcher Paula Fiet discovered that underdeveloped short-term memory may be to blame for some students' problems with mastering concepts in math and reading."[45]

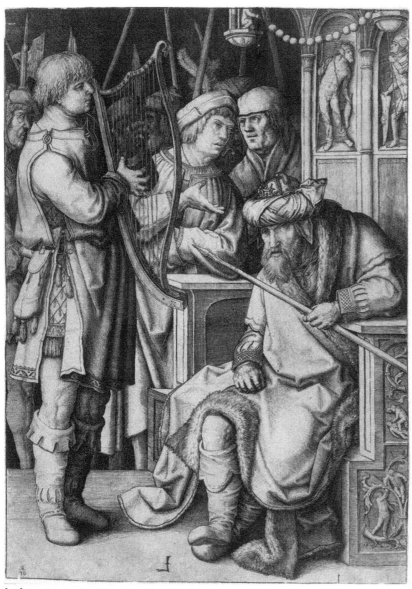

[45] David playing Harp for King Saul

"Because music was thought to have a therapeutic effect, the king summoned...David, who was renowned for his skill with the harp.

David soothed the troubled king. David's pleasing performances would eventually lead to him succeeding Saul as the king of Israel. "Courtesy of The Art Institute of Chicago."...David would play his harp [and] Saul would relax and feel better, and the evil spirit would go away.

I Samuel 16:23

Calligraphy

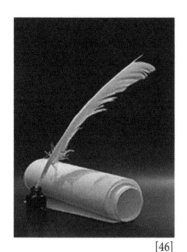

Ella was a gifted artist, singer, and musician—a renaissance woman without question. I did not need to seek her recommendation of an activity to help me fill the agonizing emptiness of my continuing isolation. She frequently had demonstrated this fascinating and purposeful skill within her hobby of scrapbooking and calligraphy.

Several times on occasions of joy and sorrow, my family received her personalized cards and [46] notes that were lavish works of art flawlessly customized to match the mood and circumstances. Her flowing expressions made incredible impressions especially because of her effort to individualize the messages for us alone.

I had observed this old style writing in Bibles, diaries, journals, and logbooks in my grandmother's primitive collectibles, but never had the will to learn how to do it until this occasion. Subsequently, I discovered practicing this beautiful writing provides multiple benefits, particularly related to relieving stress and improving mental health.

Calligraphy activates the motor areas of the brain, which include the cerebral cortex, the basal ganglia, and cerebellum. At the same time, it engages the language portion of the brain. It is meditative, relaxing, helps develop fine motor skills, and memory retention.

Special chiseled calligraphy pens are available now in office supply stores and the internet, but what did our forefathers use? The wing feathers primarily from crows, geese, and turkeys have been used since medieval times to create writing quills for record-keepers and scribes. They would split the feather at its point, which would retain a fair amount of homemade ink when dipped into small glass containers known as wells.

Skilled orthographers used them to write in this beautiful hand-writing using fancy, decorative penmanship, somewhat like an artist painting a portrait. In recent decades calligraphy has been revived and utilized in many impressive ways.

Thirty lettering experts in calligraphy *skills.com* it is "a set of skills and techniques for positioning and inscribing words so they show in-tegrity, harmony, some sort of ancestry, rhythm and creative fire."

I plan to use this skill to write personal notes of affection, apprecia-tion, love, and sympathy in the future.

Throughout the last half of June up until July 2, 2020, I continued to pick the minds of dozens of resource persons about ways and means of addressing solitary confinement. Somewhat like the conversation between Alice and the Cheshire Cat in the Wonderland, I initially did not know where I was going with this book. However, necessity soon became the mother of invention, or as Plato phrased it in his Republic in 375 BC, "our need will be the real creator."

An article in the New York Times updated September 18, 2020, by Jonathan Corum, Katherine J. Wu, and Carl Zimmer asserts "there is no cure yet for Covid-19.[46] Even the most promising treatments to date only help certain groups of patients and await validation from further trials. The F.D.A. has not fully licensed any treatment specifically for the coronavirus. Although it has granted emergency use authorization to some treatments, their effectiveness against Covid-19 has yet to be demonstrated in large-scale, randomized clinical trials."[1]

As of September 27, 2020, a total of 32,886,465 cases have been confirmed in more than 227 countries and territories. 9,131,564 are active cases and 994,940 have resulted in death. There is little I can

---

1 A flash forward to Nov 9, 2020, breaking morning news revieled that Pfizer Pharmacuticals and it's german partner, Biotech have developed a vacine that is 90% effective in preventing infection from Covid-19. The impact remains to be seen but has no direct bearing on this narritive.

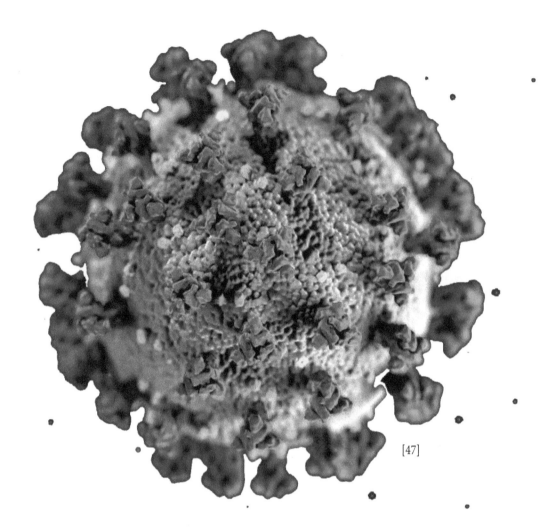

[47]

contribute to the physical treatment and cure of COVID-19.

Therefore, the ways and means by which I found emotional and mental relief is the compelling message in this book. I am excited to continue sharing them in the interest of others coping with depression and stress. None were original with me. I learned more from well-informed experts about "what's what" in terms of common sense and practical knowledge in three weeks than I had learned in 14 years of formal education.

Art Therapy

My research into stress-alleviating activities introduced me to Pablo Picasso, a Spanish painter and sculptor. He was one of the most influential and unusual artists of the 20th century even as evidenced by the length of his name: Pablo Diego José Francisco de Paula Juan Nepomuceno María de los Remedios Cipriano de la Santísima Trinidad Ruiz y Picasso.

His paintings frequently depict sadness, depression, and isolation. This woman shown as an inmate staring at her cell wall, portrays exactly how I felt throughout my confinement.

His most famous saying directed me to Art Therapy and the aesthetic pleasure it provided.

"*ART WASHES AWAY FROM THE SOUL THE DUST OF EVERYDAY LIFE.*" [47]

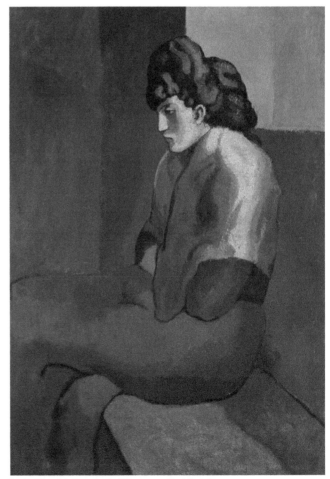

[48] *The Melancholy Woman*—Pablo Picasso

Several of my family members are artistically inclined. My sister, Natalie, especially is talented and is an Art Education major in college. I asked her and my step-mom, Cynthia, and others for their recommendations for idle time activities that would help me address the boredom. They were all-in with art related suggestions.

Fortunately, I found a project in waiting. My grandmother's six metal American flag yard signs had rusted and needed to be repainted. I ordered by curbside pickup the paint—red, white, and blue, sheets of course and fine sandpaper, brushes, and mineral spirits to clean up.

The American flag painting project was also meaningful to my Granddad. Even though it involved only miniature yard flags, as a U. S. Navy veteran and staunch patriot, he insists they symbolically are to be respected. "In 1782, Charles Thompson, the secretary of the Continental Congress, described the red in our Country's Great Seal as representing hardiness and valor; the white, purity and innocence; and the blue, vigilance, perseverance and justice. Five years later, these same representations were believed to have been assigned to the colors of the flag." [48]

When misguided souls dishonor and disrespect *Old Glory* and our National Anthem, tears come to Granddad's eyes. He agonizes over the one million killed in America's wars who cannot rise to defend its principles once again—even to protect the right of those who wish to insult our badges of honor.

Ninety-seven year old Bob Dole, a retired congressman, senator, statesman, and wounded warrior of World War II is helped out of his wheelchair to salute the flag draped casket of former President George H. W. Bush. [49]

This supreme act of patriotism and homage is especially significant upon considering that Dole was severely injured in Italy while helping a fellow soldier. He was hit by a German bullet which injured his collar-

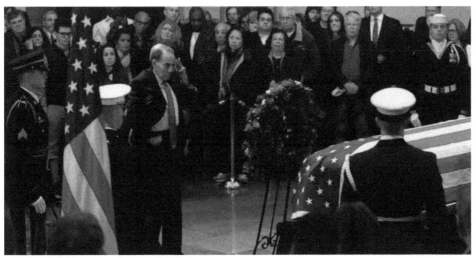

[49] Bob Dole salutes Bush casket

bone and spine paralyzing him from the neck down. Dole received two Purple Hearts and two Bronze Stars[48] for valor among other honors for his sacrifices on behalf of our country. It touched me to my core, especially after learning in the preceding that in 1782, Charles Thompson, the secretary of the Continental Congress, described the red in our flag as representing valor. Unfortunately, some people just don't get it! My sentiments are best expressed by Billy Ray and Cindy Cyrus in their hit, *Some Gave All!*[50]

Granddad, you can rest assured I never will disrespect our Anthem nor our flag, and principles for which they stand: hardiness, innocence, justice, perseverance, purity, valor and vigilance. It would be the most shameful and ungrateful act of defiance I could ever imagine. Never!

[50]

Soon, I will have Grandmother's tin yard flags sanded, painted, and looking like new again. For the moment, I need a tissue, there is a lump in my throat and my eyes are watering.

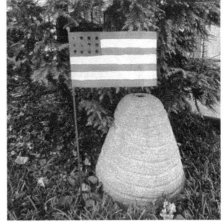

[50a]

...Praise the power that hath made and preserv'd us a nation!
Then conquer we must, when our cause it is just,
And this be our motto - "In God is our trust,"
And the star-spangled banner in triumph shall wave
O'er the land of the free and the home of the brave.[51]

The Star-Spangled Banner—Francis Scott Key

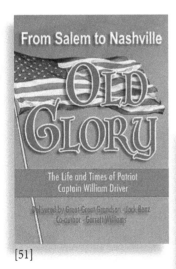

[51]

I am grateful to acknowledge that my Granddad and Great Aunt volunteered their services as editor and graphics designer on this COVID-19 narrative. They also collaborated with author Jack Benz to help produce *Old Glory From Salem to Nashville*, the Life and Times of Captain William Driver, Nashville's legendary patriot, who gave the name, *Old Glory* to the American Flag.

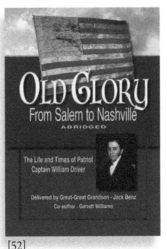

[52]

How Owning a Dog or Cat Can Reduce Stress

Elizabeth Scott writing in the website,[52] *Very Well Mind* tells how having a pet can help lessen stress in the following ways:

1. Improves one's mood
2. Helps control blood pressure
3. Encourages one to get moving
4. Helps with social support
5. Staves off loneliness and provides unconditional love.

"Research shows that pets can provide excellent social support, stress relief, and other health benefits—perhaps more than people. It is virtually impossible to stay in a bad mood when a pair of loving puppy eyes meets yours, or when a super-soft cat rubs against your hand [or leg].

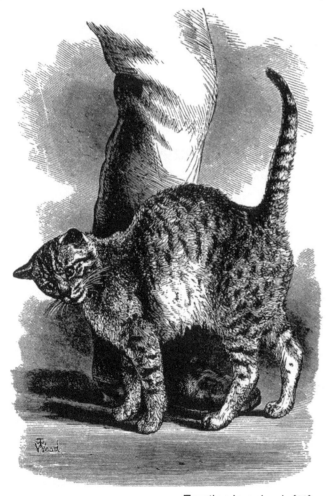

Emotion in animals [53]

"Yes, it's true. While ACE inhibiting drugs can generally reduce blood pressure, they aren't effective in controlling spikes in blood pressure due to stress and tension. Research has concluded since the mid-1980's that there are positive physiological effects, particularly lowered blood pressure, to petting dogs and social interaction with companion animals. The actual act of petting the dog appeared to be the major component of the so-called pet effect.

"Whether we walk our dogs because they need it, or are more likely to enjoy a walk when we have companionship, dog owners do spend more time walking than non-pet owners, at least if we live in an urban setting.

"Most people with dogs will likely say that they enjoy their walks more because of their pets' companionship, and perhaps even the feeling of being part of a community of other pet lovers. Because exercise is good for stress management and overall health, owning a dog can be credited.

"When we're out walking, having a dog with us can make us more approachable and give people a reason to stop and talk. The increased number of people we meet allows us to expand our network of friends and acquaintances, which also has excellent stress management benefits.

"Pets can be there for us in ways that people can't. They can offer love and companionship and enjoy comfortable silences, keep secrets, and are excellent snugglers.

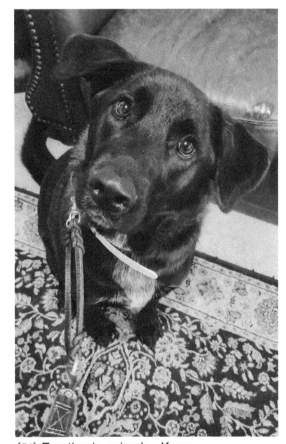

"Also, they could be the best antidote to loneliness. One study found that nursing home residents reported less loneliness when visited by dogs alone than when they spent time with dogs and other people. All these benefits can reduce the amount of stress people experience in response to social isolation and lack of social support.

"Pets Can Sometimes Reduce Stress Even More Than People. While

[54] Emotion in animals - Knox

we all know the power of talking about our problems with a good friend who is also a good listener; research shows that spending time with a pet may be even better.

"Another study showed that people experienced less stress when their pets were with them when conducting a stressful task than when a supportive friend or spouse was present. This may be partially because pets don't judge us; they just love us.

"It's important to realize that owning a pet isn't for everyone. Pets do come with additional work and responsibility, which can bring its own stress. However, for most people, the benefits of having a pet outweigh the drawbacks. Having a furry best friend can reduce stress in your life and bring you support when times get tough."

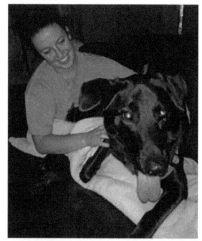

[55]

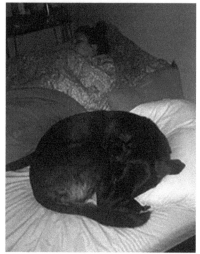

[56]

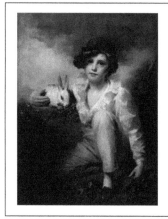

[57]

My great-grandparents had two boys, including my granddad. Treating animals with love and kindness was engrained early on and reinforced by framed prints of animals throughout their home. Perhaps I inherited this tendency.

Boy and Rabbit by Henry Raeburn

The Covid-19 experience has made me more mindful than ever of the healing benefit my dogs have provided.

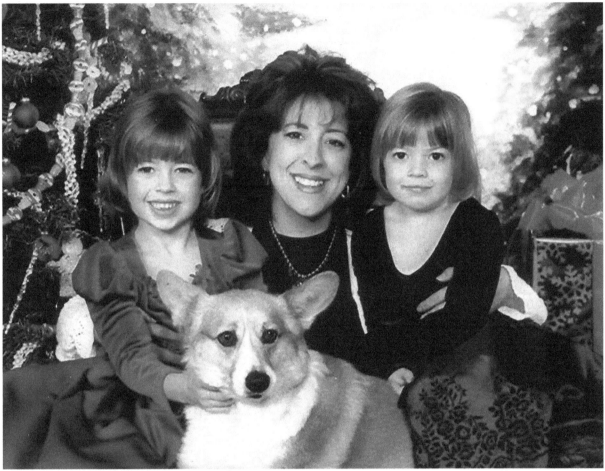

[58] Ginger, Carol, Natalie, and Claire

This 2002 family Christmas portrait reinforces the value of Claire in our family circle. My mom is holding my sister and me as we caress our dog. She was a point of contact to convey her unconditional love, even while crippled. She could not stand or move her rear legs but would drag herself by her two front legs to comfort us and receive a pat.

The emotional support animals provide is so hallowed that, under Federal Law,[53] Emotional Support Animals must have access to apartments even with a no-pet policy and exempt from pet-related fees.

Mr. Lucky's Buddies

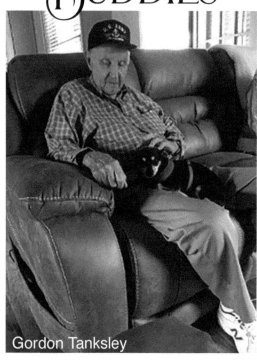

Gordon Tanksley

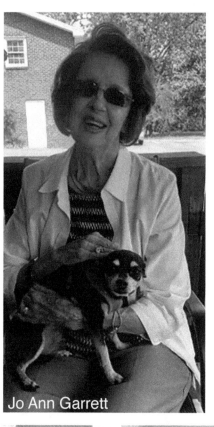

Jo Ann Garrett

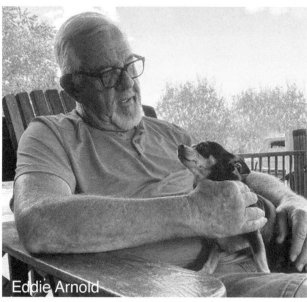

Eddie Arnold

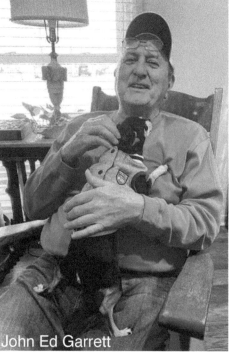

John Ed Garrett

[59]

WHAT ABOUT ME FOR A BUDDY?

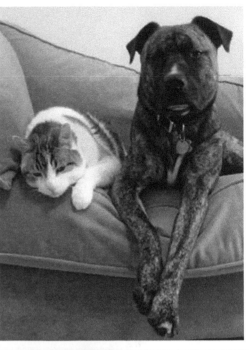

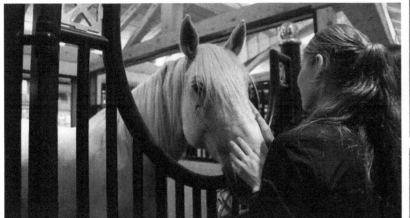

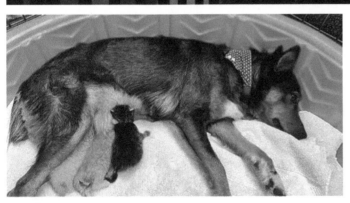

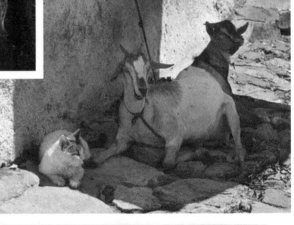

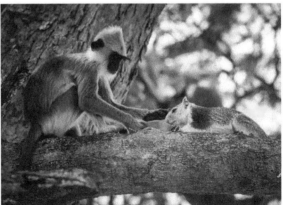

[60]

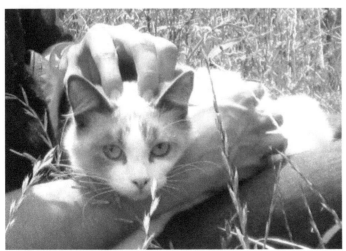

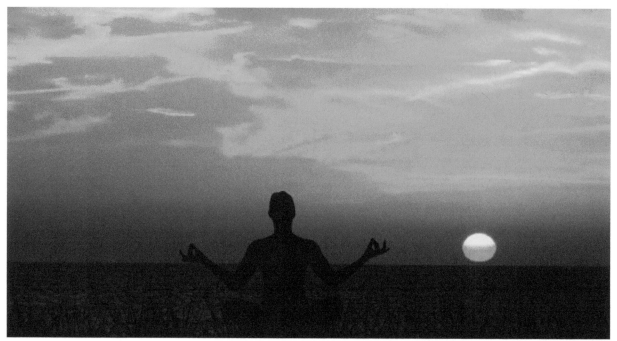

Yoga and Aerobics

The *Harvard Publishing* Mental Health letter updated on May 9, 2018, says, "many patients dealing with depression, anxiety, or stress, may find Yoga to be a very appealing way to better manage symptoms. Indeed, Yoga's scientific study demonstrates that mental and physical health are not just closely allied, but are essentially equivalent.[54]

"Yoga could be considered an all-round exercise that will take care of the body, mind, and soul, according to Tiwari (Hindu Brahmins) who said practicing it has been known to be beneficial for all ages.[55] Yoga is for health, harmony, and happiness, he stressed, and one can achieve a mindfulness and thoughtless state practicing Yoga."

Numerous health-related periodicals such as *Harvard Health* highlight the mental and emotional benefits of aerobic exercise provides neurochemically. "Exercise reduces levels of the body's stress hormones, such as adrenaline and cortisol. It also stimulates the production of endorphins, the chemicals in the brain that are the body's natural painkillers and mood elevators."

Link to a 20-minute workout:
https://www.youtube.com/watch?v=WXUCoAM7eqw

According to the Cleveland Clinic, aerobic (cardio exercises) provide cardiovascular conditioning.[56] "The American Heart Association recommends a minimum of 30 minutes of cardiovascular exercise 5 to 7 days per week. They emphasize not to forget warm-up, cool-down and stretching exercises in your aerobic exercise session. Swimming, walking, running, jogging, stair climbing, dancing, skiing, skipping, and hiking.

Benefits of aerobic exercise:
- It improves cardiovascular conditioning.
- It decreases the risk of heart disease.
- It helps lower blood pressure.
- It increases HDL (good) cholesterol.
- It helps control blood sugar.
- Assists in weight management and weight loss.
- Improves lung function and decreases resting heart rate."

Movies

Dr. Gary Solomon, an author of two books on cinema therapy, says "we should choose movies with themes that mirror our current problems or situation. They trigger emotional releases that can have a cathartic effect and make it easier to express our emotions. This can be invaluable during counseling as well as in real life.[57]

"Movies bring us a sense of relief, even if they stress us out first. Watching something suspenseful releases cortisol—the stress hormone—in the brain, followed by dopamine, which produces pleasure feelings. We are transported to a different time and place and give our brains a much-needed rest from the usual."

In addition to documentaries, *Bright Side YouTube Channel* ranks the following 15 as some of the most memorable movies about life-changing journeys. They are inspirational and especially comforting to those in quarantine.

1. A Perfect Getaway
2. The Edge
3. Taken 2
4. Point Break, 2015
5. Cast Away
6. Into the Wild
7. Leap Year
8. The Painted Veil
9. Kon-Tiki
10. The Physician
11. The Best Exotic Marigold Hotel
12. Midnight in Paris
13. To Rome with Love
14. The Darjeeling Limited
15. The Good Dinosaur

All-time Best 100 Movies

Sources include Amazon, Goodwill stores, libraries, Netflix, Redbox, YouTube, and other streaming services. They can be viewed on computers, DVD players, TVs, smartphones, and tablets.

Highest Grossing film of all times.

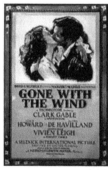

[62]

The 100 best films ever, according to the American Film Institute.

RANK	MOVIE TITLE	YEAR	RANK	MOVIE TITLE	YEAR
1	CITIZEN KANE	1941	25	TO KILL A MOCKINGBIRD	1962
2	THE GODFATHER	1972	26	MR. SMITH WASHINGTON	1939
3	CASABLANCA	1942	27	HIGH NOON	1952
4	RAGING BULL	1980	28	ALL ABOUT EVE	1950
5	SINGIN' IN THE RAIN	1952	29	DOUBLE INDEMNITY	1944
6	GONE WITH THE WIND	1939	30	APOCALYPSE NOW	1979
7	LAWRENCE OF ARABIA	1962	31	THE MALTESE FALCON	1941
8	SCHINDLER'S LIST	1993	32	THE GODFATHER PART II	1974
9	VERTIGO	1958	33	CUCKOO'S NEST	1975
10	THE WIZARD OF OZ	1939	34	SNOW WHITE & DWARFS	1937
11	CITY LIGHTS	1931	35	ANNIE HALL	1977
12	THE SEARCHERS	1956	36	BRIDGE ON RIVER KWAI	1957
13	STAR WARS	1977	37	BEST YEARS OUR LIVES	1946
14	PSYCHO	1960	38	TREASURE SIERRA	1948
15	2001: A SPACE ODYSSEY	1968	39	DR. STRANGELOVE	1964
16	SUNSET BOULEVARD	1950	40	THE SOUND OF MUSIC	1965
17	THE GRADUATE	1967	41	KING KONG	1933
18	THE GENERAL	1927	42	BONNIE AND CLYDE	1967
19	ON THE WATERFRONT	1954	43	MIDNIGHT COWBOY	1969
20	IT'S A WONDERFUL LIFE	1946	44	PHILADELPHIA STORY	1940
21	CHINATOWN	1974	45	SHANE	1953
22	SOME LIKE IT HOT	1959	46	HAPPENED ONE NIGHT	1934
23	THE GRAPES OF WRATH	1940	47	A STREETCAR DESIRE	1951
24	EXTRA-TERRESTRIAL	1982	48	REAR WINDOW	1954

RANK	MOVIE TITLE	YEAR	RANK	MOVIE TITLE	YEAR
49	INTOLERANCE	1916	76	FORREST GUMP	1994
50	THE LORD OF THE RING	2001	75	HEAT OF THE NIGHT	1967
51	WEST SIDE STORY	1961	77	ALL PRESIDENT'S MEN	1976
52	TAXI DRIVER	1976	78	MODERN TIMES	1936
53	THE DEER HUNTER	1978	79	THE WILD BUNCH	1969
54	M*A*S*H	1970	80	THE APARTMENT	1960
55	NORTH BY NORTHWEST	1959	81	SPARTACUS	1960
56	JAWS	1975	82	SUNRISE	1927
57	ROCKY	1976	83	TITANIC	1997
58	THE GOLD RUSH	1925	84	EASY RIDER	1969
59	NASHVILLE	1975	85	A NIGHT AT THE OPERA	1935
60	DUCK SOUP	1933	86	PLATOON	1986
61	SULLIVAN'S TRAVELS	1941	87	12 ANGRY MEN	1957
62	AMERICAN GRAFFITI	1973	88	BRINGING UP BABY	1938
63	CABARET	1972	89	THE SIXTH SENSE	1999
64	NETWORK	1976	90	SWING TIME	1936
65	THE AFRICAN QUEEN	1951	91	SOPHIE'S CHOICE	1982
66	RAIDERS LOST ARK	1981	92	GOODFELLAS	1990
67	AFD VIRGINIA WOOLF	1966	93	FRENCH CONNECTION	1971
68	UNFORGIVEN	1992	94	PULP FICTION	1994
69	TOOTSIE	1982	95	LAST PICTURE SHOW	1971
70	A CLOCKWORK ORANGE	1971	96	DO THE RIGHT THING	1989
71	SAVING PRIVATE RYAN	1998	97	BLADE RUNNER	1982
72	SHANK REDEMPTION	1994	98	YANKEE DOODLE	1942
73	BUTCH AND THE KID	1969	99	TOY STORY	1995
74	THE SILENCE LAMBS	1991	100	BEN-HUR	1959

Games

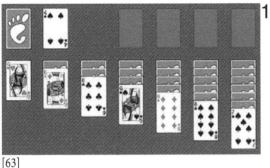

[63]

1. Solitaire card games can be played alone with real decks or using online apps from Google Play and the Apple App Store. Its popularity is such that it has reached more than 119 million players, and can be learned in five minutes. It is a logic-based cognitive game that sharpens the mind using mathematical deductions to draw conclusions.

2. Shanghai Mahjong is a matching tile game with over 10 million electronic versions sold. It is easy to learn and provides excellent mental exercise. Researchers at the University of Georgia found that Mahjong may reduce depression rates among middle-aged and older Chinese.[58]

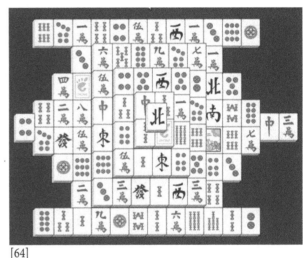

[64]

3. Computer, phone, and tablet games often are age-related. This connects resources linking to 2,500 DOS games. https://lifehacker.com/five-best-resources-for-free-games

4. Lego - This is a Danish toy production company based in Billund, Denmark. The primary toy consists mostly of interlocking plastic bricks. The Lego Group became the world's largest toy company by revenue, with sales amounting to $2.1 billion in the

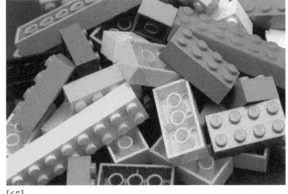

[65]

U.S., surpassing Mattel, which had $1.9 billion in sales.

Lego develops problem-solving and mathematical thinking.

Genealogy

In my new found love for reading, I was drawn to the domains of philosophy and religion. Three questions continued to emerge for me to answer: Who am I, where am I going, and why? These three genealogy-related questions are also the three that form the basis of all the world's major religions.

Family history, as revealed to me by relatives, became my primary resource to begin my search. My great-great maternal grandfather shared an interesting story in this regard. When my mother and her brother were born, questions of ancestry became of interest to Granddad. He asked his father the name of his father, grandfather, and about their family heritage. Shockingly, my great-great-grandfather did not know the name of his own father, who had died when he was only six months old.

There were no written records whatsoever, but an elderly aunt offered a clue, which led to my grandfather finding a country cemetery holding the missing link. He discovered several hundred ancestors using the tombstone information, state archives resources, and the world's leading online research company, Ancestry.com. Ultimately, his work reunited our family with cousins worldwide.

Genealogy officially is the study of families and the history of their lineages. It is beneficial in several ways but is incomparable for those quarantined as an activity to combat idleness and loneliness. Further, it carries over as a worthwhile lifetime on-going study beyond

COVID-19. It is highly addictive in a whole-some sense but equally provides a joyful journey investigating thousands of ancestors' lifetimes and their influences on one's past, present, and future.

I'm fortunate that a lot of my family information is already researched and recorded. Census records are a great place to start verifying location, name, age, and relation to the household's head. Early census records give very little information, but 1850 provides much more.

According to the 72-year rule, the National Archives releases census records to the general public 72 years after Census Day. As a result, the 1930 records were released on April 1, 2002,[60] the 1940 records on April 2, 1912, and the 1950 records will be released in April 2022. This will enable a whole new generation to be added to many family trees.

One's public tree on the web will offer suggestions of records and people to add to the tree. Photographs are a bonus to bring a family tree to life. Also, family history genealogical data is available for free at state and local archives. Ancestry.com and other online services offer a two-week trial period before requiring payment.

Newspapers.com is a for-pay service but offers a great variety of information from advertisements, social events, politics, news, and obituaries. It is a very entertaining activity in itself.

Findagrave.com often provides photographs of the headstones, birth and death dates, and some biographical information attached.

For a fee, *Fold3.com* will help find a relative's military service record.

Follow this link to the 25 best genealogy related websites: https://www.familytreemagazine.com/premium/25-best-genealogy-websites-for-beginners/

Made-up Games

In addition to the numerous activities suggested by family and friends, my eyes were opened wider through personal internet searches. They literally linked to millions of individualized and small group activities, including the 1920s kissing game of chance known as "Spin the Bottle." Accordingly, I utilized the spinning concept to create a traveling game that transforms the study of geography, history, and cultures from a boring activity to one that is fun, enlightening, and, most importantly, time-consuming for those in confinement. Fittingly, I named it "Spin the Globe."

A basic globe, internet access, and an active imagination combine to provide hours of entertainment and volumes of knowledge for participants. The game involves taking imaginary trips beginning with spinning the globe and randomly stopping it with the index finger to identify an unplanned destination. The ultimate goal is to return from the trip well-informed about the locale and

[66]

92

general knowledge useful in any educational context and enlightened conversation. There is no set agenda, so whatever appeals to one's curiosity or interest becomes the narrative. Somewhat like dominoes toppling in sequence, each new bit of information multiplies to further enlightenment—one tidbit becomes two, two becomes four, etc.

For example, the result of one of my most interesting spinning trips placed my index finger directly on the city of Istanbul, Turkey—a far-away place with a strange-sounding name.[1]

My primary information-gathering resources were internet search engines such as Bing, Google, and Yahoo. Google's video-sharing platform, YouTube, by far, was the most amazing and fulfilling. My virtual trip began with a map from an encyclopedia. The illustration below reveals Turkey as a Middle East country strangely occupying two continents, Asia and Europe. They are separated by the Bosporus, which is the world's narrowest strait connecting two water bodies for international navigation. It links the Black Sea with the Sea of Marmara and, by extension, through other straits, seas, and the Atlantic Ocean enables ship navigation from America's East Coast all the way to Russia's West Coast entirely by water.

I immediately began increasing my vocabulary as I encountered unfamiliar words. For example, as used in the Bosporus Strait, the word "strait" describing a waterway separating two landmasses, is different from the same-sounding, "straight" in my vocabulary, describing a uniform line without bends or curves. Nevertheless, "strait" is a new word for me. Furthermore, the analogy to domino toppling linked me to another new word, isthmus. Whereas a strait separates two land bodies, the opposite is true of an isthmus, which separates two water bodies.

---

1 "Far Away Places" is an American popular song written by Joan Whitney and Alex Kramer and published in 1948. Willie Nelson and Sheryl Crow introduced me to an enchanting remake.

Isthmus of Panama

For example, the narrowest part of Panama separating the Caribbean Sea and the Pacific Ocean is called the *Isthmus of Panama*. It is not to be confused with the canal. However, it is noteworthy while viewing the area that about 40 ships a day pass through the Panama Canal, saving up to 8,000 water miles, otherwise avoiding having to round South America.

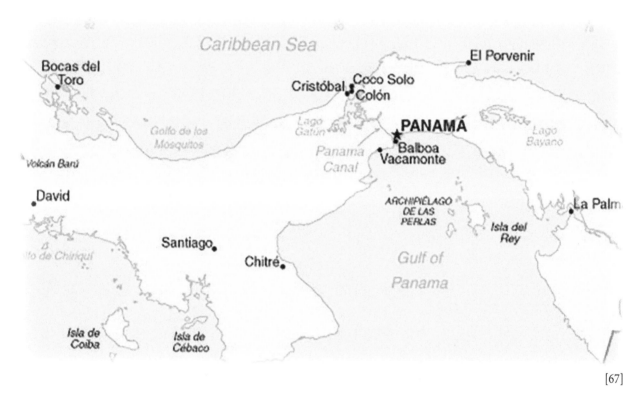

[67]

Istanbul and the Bosporus
-A city of over 15,000,000 residents

My virtual vacation to Istanbul was a mind-boggling experience that captured my attention for days. To describe the indescribable is as impossible as its definition. Perhaps I can help set the backdrop by sharing some previews. Still, to grasp the significance of the incredible revelations found in one of the world's largest and most unique cities, one must visit it virtually or in person. Virtual traveling is the only option

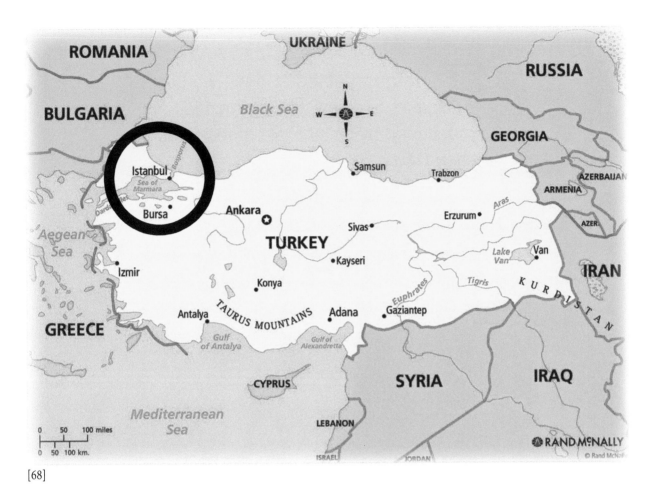

[68]

open to those quarantined, and I urge you to take this trip to sample the value of combating isolation with my "Spin the Globe" activity.

YouTube linked me to hundreds of documentaries, images, visual walking tours, and videos portraying Istanbul's culture, economics, geography, government, history, and religions.[61] The snippets to follow are examples of my virtual trip's highlights, which helped cure my loneliness.

About 300 A.D., Roman Emperor Constantine founded Constantinople on the site of the former city, Byzantium; it functioned as the capital of the Eastern Roman Empire. Rome was the capital of the Western Empire. Constantine had converted to Christianity and, in 313 A.D., granted religious freedom throughout the Empire. In 380 A.D., Emperor Theodosius made Nicene Christianity the official religion.[62]

Hagia Sophia

The current Hagia Sophia was completed in 537 A.D. by Emperor Justinian and served as the largest cathedral in the world for nearly one thousand years until Spain's Seville Cathedral in 1507. In the religious context, Turkey is mentioned by its biblical names throughout the book of *Acts* in the *Christian Bible.*

The Muslim conquest of Constantinople occurred in 1453 and resulted in the city becoming the capital of the Ottoman (Turkish) Empire under Sultan Mehmed II—The Conqueror. Mehmed II subsequently turned the Hagia Sophia into a Turkish mosque, rebuilt the destroyed city, and created an atmosphere of tolerance for Christians and Jews

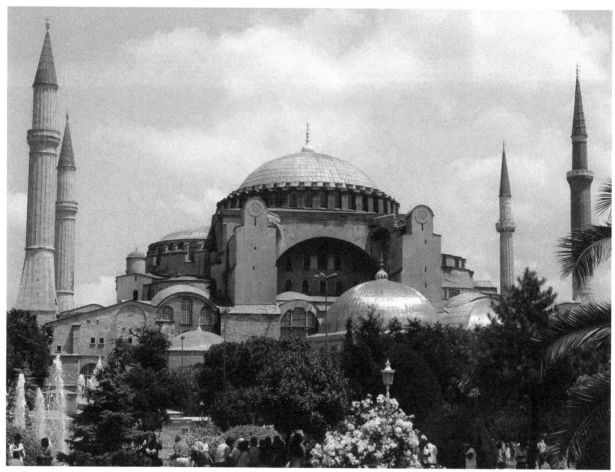

[69]

alongside the new and predominant Muslim culture.[63] The inclusiveness is evidenced in the 2000 census listing 2691 mosques, 123 active churches, and 20 active synagogues. Istanbul became the city's new name in 1930.

Notice the spire towers on top of the mosque. They are known as minarets from which the Muslim faithful are called to prayer five times a day.

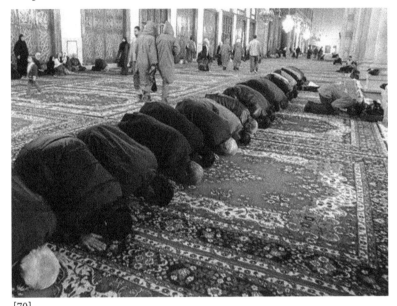
[70]

Sajdah
Prayer Position
Although Turkish is its most widely spoken language, English is a close second.

There are over 4,000 religions globally, and Turkey is home to all three of the so-called great revealed religions—those not arrived by natural reason alone. They are Judaism, Christianity, and Islam; however, 99% of Turkey's people today are Muslim.[64] Again, the domino effect led me to study all the world's greatest religions.

The 20 largest religions are:

Christianity *(2.1 billion)*
Islam *(1.3 billion)*
Nonreligious (Secular/Agnostic/Atheist) *(1.1 billion)*
Hinduism *(900 million)*
Chinese traditional religion *(394 million)*
Buddhism *(376 million)*
Primal-indigenous (300 million)
African traditional and Diasporic *(100 million)*
Sikhism *(23 million)*
Juche *(19 million)*
Spiritism (15 million)
Judaism *(14 million)*
Bahai *(7 million)*
Jainism *(4.2 million)*
Shinto *(4 million)*
Cao Dai *(4 million)*
Zoroastrianism *(2.6 million)*
Tenrikyo *(2 million)*
Neo-Paganism *(1 million)*
Unitarian-Universalism *(800,000)*[65]

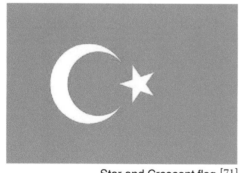

Star and Crescent flag [71]

The star and crescent flags displayed throughout Istanbul typically is the international symbol of the Islamic faith.

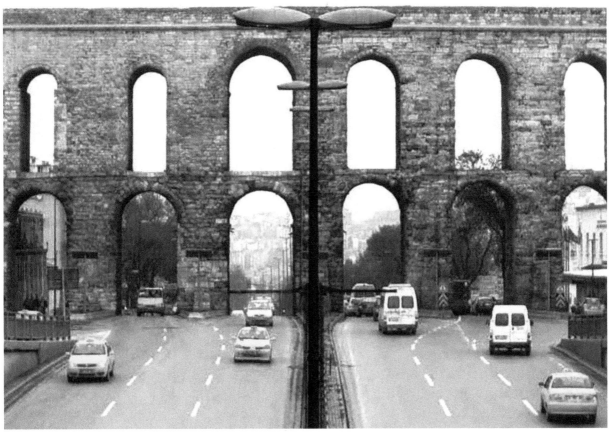

[72]

Aqueduct of Valens

This aqueduct was completed in 368 AD during the reign of Roman Emperor Valens. It essentially is a man-made stream that conducts water downhill from the natural sources to the destination by gravity.

   Although virtual, it is an amazing experienc to visit Istanbul via You-Tube and look upon the same structure that other eyes saw 1,652 years ago.

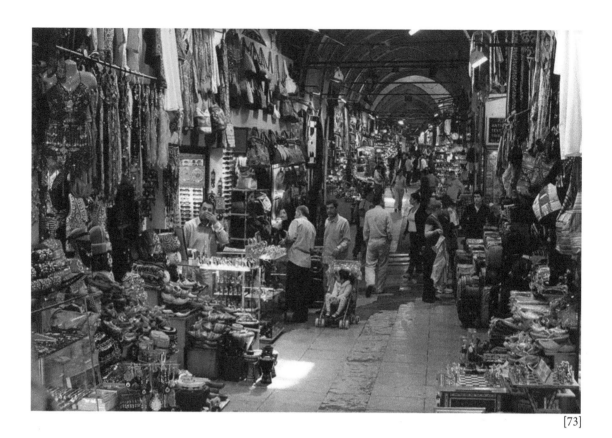

[73]

This image gives a glimpse of what I saw virtually in the world's largest and most visited tourist attraction—The Grand Bazaar in Istanbul. It is contained in 61 covered streets within more than 4,000 shops attracting over a quarter million visitors daily. Many amazing live videos are available on YouTube —a must see (in person or virtually!)

Turkish Bath

I had heard of Turkish baths but never understood their meaning or purpose. This virtual exposure to the widespread presence of Turkish bathhouses or Hammams throughout Istanbul enlightened me. The experience is a popular luxury for the locals and a must-do for first-time tourists.

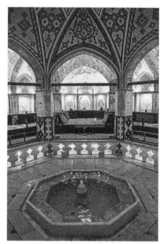

[74]

The use of steam, hot and cold water, aromatherapy, deep scrubbing techniques with unique exfoliating soaps, and massages leave the pores soft and hydrated. Turkish baths relieve sore muscles, improve blood circulation by dilating blood vessels, and eliminate chest congestion. It is as popular as going to the hairdresser, nail shop or barber shop.

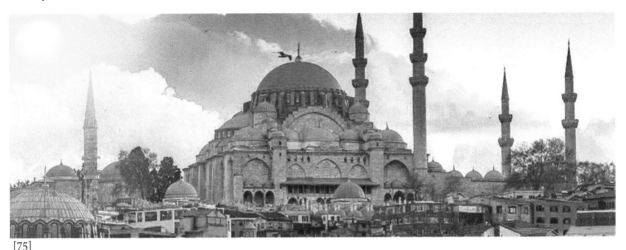

[75]

The Blue Mosque

The Sultan Armed Mosque, because of its thousands of hand-painted blue tiles inside and blue lighting outside, also is known as the Blue

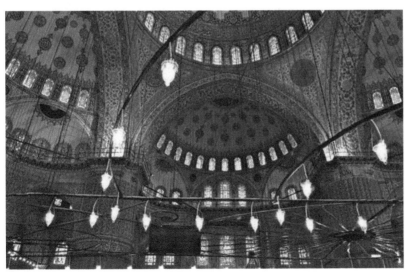

[76]

Mosque. It was constructed between 1609 and 1616 and is one of Istanbul's most popular tourist attractions.[66]

My virtual trip to the city occupied my time for several days and was an adventure of a lifetime without ever leaving my bedroom. It truly is one of the oldest and most beautiful cities in the world. I invite all who are isolated and have access to You-Tube to enjoy a vicarious exotic vacation there along with the other top ten cities I visited via my "spin the globe game." They are:

1- Kyoto, Japan.
2- Dubrovnik, Croatia.
3- St. Petersburg, Russia.
4- Prague, Czech Republic.
5- Cape Town, South Africa.
6- Bergen, Norway.
7- Istanbul, Turkey.
8- San Francisco, United States.
9- Venice, Italy
10- San Miguel de Allende, Mexico

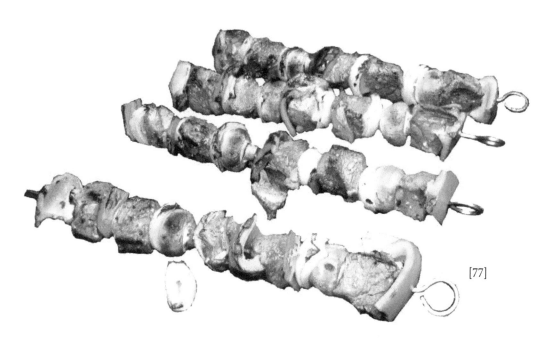

[77]

Kebab or shish kebab unquestionably is Turkey's most famous food. It is made from small cuts of marinated meat cooked and served on skewers.

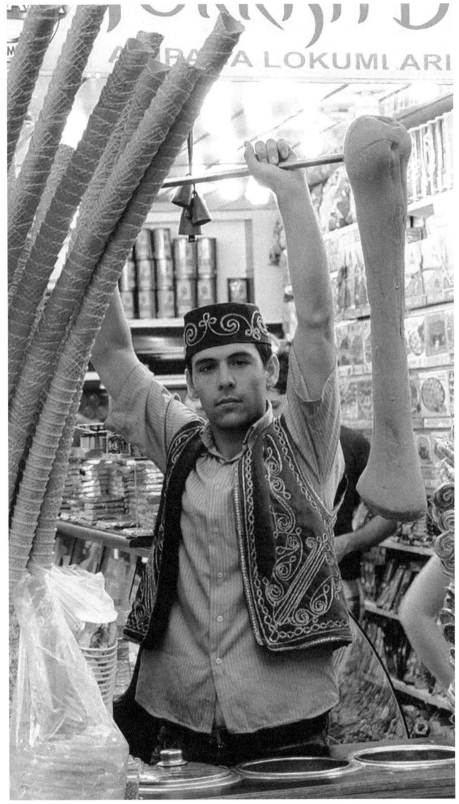

Stretchy
super cool
Turkish
ice cream
sold by a
street
vendor

[78] Donduama (Ice Cream)

LAW OF COMPOUNDING

$0.01
$0.02
$0.04
$0.08
$0.16
$0.32
$0.64
$1.28
$2.56
$5.12
$10.24
$20.48
$40.96
$81.92
$163.84
$327.68
$655.36
$1,310.72
$2,621.44
$5,242.88
$10,485.76
$20,971.52
$41,943.04
$83,886.08
$167,772.16
$335,544.32
$671,068.64
$1,342,177.28
$2,684,354.56 [79]
$5,368,709.12
$10,737,418.23
$21,474,836.46

Online Investing

There is no better use of idle time while confined than to seek knowledge and skills that build retirement income to supplement savings, company pensions, and social security. One can be entertained and informed online for hours while becoming savvy in economics. An account can be opened to serve as a resource and practice without depositing money.

In the first months of my new career, I necessarily am forced to make decisions my parents made on my behalf for more than two decades. Fortunately, in the weeks spent in confinement, I received guidance from mentors along with personal studies that prepared me to make informed decisions. I share this exciting option to encourage others in similar circumstances to consider.

Before collecting my first paycheck, I completed documents related to, of all things, retirement. I sought advice from several who were very astute, including one who actively teaches self-directed investing to rookies. He introduced to me some eye-opening concepts and practices framed in some challenging questions.

"Ginger, let's begin your crash course with two exercises and one Commandment. The first question is, would you prefer that I give you one penny doubled each day for a month, or a million dollars and just forget about the computations? In other words, the progression from day one would be 1 cent, 2, 4, 8, 16, etc. He spared me the trouble and embarrassment of making a foolish choice. The chart to the left indicates at the end of 31 days, I would have accumulated ten million, seven-hundred thirty-seven thousand, four hundred eighteen dollars and 23 cents!

"As one can see, accepting one million upfront would be a terrible choice; however, the illustration shows the magic of compound interest.

"The second exercise was for me to understand the financial *'rule of 72.'* Accordingly, the principal amount is divided by the interest rate to determine how long it will take for the money to double. There are *'rule of 72'* calculators on the internet available to quickly determine the answer, but he asked me to compute some examples for practice. Therefore, at 10% interest divided into 72, the answer would be 7.2 years for the original sum to double. Even more astounding was in the second segment of 7.2 years, the doubling was of an amount already doubled, thus resulting in quadrupling the original amount.

"The interest return on most S & P 500 index funds averages around 10% but has been as high as 29% within the past ten years. That would be an unusually rare occasion, but in that instance, the principal amount would double by dividing 72 by 29, which would be 2.4 years."

His third point, which he termed the *Commandment of Frugality*, is that I must be a good steward of my earnings by always paying myself first, 10% of all income, and investing it to be fruitful as per the Biblical parable of the talents:

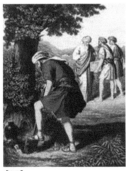

[80]

...then the man who had received one bag of gold came. Master, he said, I knew that you are a hard man...so I was afraid and went out and hid your gold in the ground. See, here is what belongs to you. His master replied, you wicked, lazy servant... you should have put my money on deposit with the bankers, so that when I returned I would have received it back with interest. So take the bag of gold and give it to the one who has ten bags. For whoever has will be given more, and they will have an abundance. Whoever does not have, even what they have will be taken from them." — Matthew 25 14-30

Although the preceding mathmatical illustrations were informative and compelling, it is ironic that my economics classes prepared me the least. In high school, I learned about the law of supply and demand, amortization, banking, borrowing, budgeting, compound interest, mortgaging, and such, but very little about investing. In fairness to my teachers, internet investing was in its relative infancy, and offline brokerage requirements were outside most students' reach. I had no idea that I could own a part of 500 of the world's wealthiest companies for around fifty dollars by purchasing only one share of a Standard & Poors index fund.

After reading several books, dozens of articles, learning from numerous successful investors, and establishing an online brokerage account, I entered a new arena—The United States Stock Exchange (NYSC)—valued at 34 trillion dollars. It is the largest stock exchange in the world, three times greater than the second in size, the Nasdaq, also a New York exchange.[67]

My grandparents bought stocks before the internet was opened to the public in 1993. They were required to transact through a broker who typically charged a $40 fee plus 1% of the cost set by the number of shares purchased. Today, the trades are executed electronically in real-time and are free of transaction charges in most instances. I found self-directed stock investing for play or real to be tremendously educational, fun, rewarding, and time-consuming in a positive way. However, it is not without risks as a result of bad decisions or unforeseen adverse circumstances.

There are dozens of reputable online brokerage firms. Many have local brick and mortar stores with agents that offer general advice but never specific recommendations to buy or sell; nor will I. It is a self-directed process; however, I will share what I learned from the advice of two of the world's most renowned investors and my investment advisor.

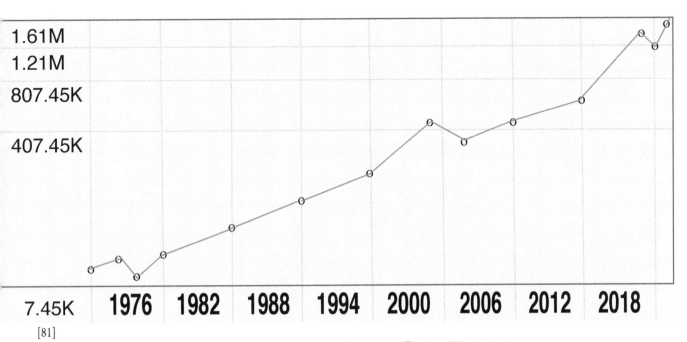

| | 1976 | 1982 | 1988 | 1994 | 2000 | 2006 | 2012 | 2018 |

1.61M
1.21M
807.45K

407.45K

7.45K

[81]

50-year chart of the S & P 500

John (Jack) Bogle, founder of Vanguard Investments, and Warren Buffett, founder of Berkshire Hathaway, and the world's 7th richest man at 68 billion dollars, are my mentors. Both assert that financial independence begins with the "paying yourself first" principle, the same as stated by my financial advisor. This simple strategy means setting aside the first 10 percent of every dollar earned for savings and investments.

The most straightforward and efficient investment strategy is to buy and hold all the nation's publicly held businesses." As previously mentioned, a S & P 500 index fund accomplishes that. The experts emphasize that less than 5% of professional advisory services charging fees can beat this strategy.

$15,000 invested in Vanguard Brokerage Firm's (500) index fund in 1976 was valued in 2006 at $461,771. The magic of compounding interest explains this phenomenal growth because interest paid on the principal amount compounds itself monthly. The S&P 500 has averaged between 8% and 10% annualized return since 1957.

As previously mentioned, The rule of 72 is applied to estimate the number of years required to double the invested money. A tax-free Roth retirement account is what the experts say should be our first investment and is currently limited to $6,000 in contributions per year.

At a 10% return for computational ease, 72/10 = 7.2 years for the original $6,000 to become $12,000. Continuing for another 7.2 years, the $12,000 becomes $24,000 because a double has been doubled. A third such sequence would double that which already has been doubled or quadrupled as follows: $6m-$12m-$24m-$48m-$96m. The original 6m increases exponentially by 2, 4, 8,16 times, etc.

Hypothetically, it would take 28.8 years (4x7.2) to complete the sequence, i.e., the sum of the doubled amounts doubling three more times. Consequently, the original $6,000 has become $96,000. If one began this tax-free Roth investment in the S & P 500 index at age 31, they would be approximately 59 and one-half years old and eligible to start withdrawing without paying income tax.

Consider further, a person can begin a new $6,000 Roth every year as long as they are employed. Contributions can be made in one lump sum or monthly, which "dollar-cost" averages the high and low purchases. Therefore, after reaching retirement age in 30 years, one could withdraw $96,000 in supplemental income at $800 per month for a year irrespective of company retirement plans and social security.

This hypothetical $800 per month tax-free income would continue for 30 years until age 92. Again, this is a supplement and doesn't factor against social security, company pensions, and other investments.

I sometimes am challenged by mathematics, but with tutoring and practice, I have been able to grasp this concept, process, and proceed with its implementation. When I scratch my head over a complex issue, my parents tell me, "if it were easy, everybody could do it, then the accomplishment would lose its value."

Considering all the "things to do" activities I have mentioned to combat boredom and idleness in quarantine, learning self-directed investing is the most worthwhile and financially rewarding.

There is one additional component to this phenomenal investment in my future. A practical, old-timer mentor suggested that I utilize the banks and credit card services to contribute free money to help pay for my stock purchases. I will share this amazing system and strategy he taught me.

Credit Cards-Windfall or Nemesis?

I often have heard, "you can't teach old dogs new tricks." The saying does not mention that incredible new tricks are available to young dogs from the old dogs' experiences and wisdom.

Uncle Butch was an old dog, unconventional character. There was drama in just about everything he said and did. Accordingly, when he told me how I legally could utilize human nature to get banks and credit card companies' to contribute to my stock purchases. I was shocked.

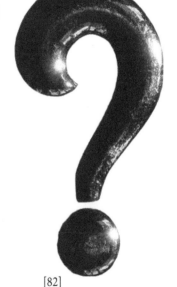

[82]

He described his plan in a manner as though it were a deep, dark secret. The setting was my favorite restaurant, where we were celebrating my birthday. Social distancing was well-established, so no other diners could hear our conversation's content or distinguish a single word of his softly delivered comments. While waiting for our order, he mysteriously leaned forward, slowly glancing left to right as if confirming that no spy was hiding thereabouts attempting to overhear us. It all was a part of his mantra to capture my concentration and interest.

He opened our session, presenting me with a "recovery gift" in the form of a credit card in my name containing a generous deposit to add to my stock account. A major bank had issued a card with rewards I could use to help pay for my stocks free of charge. Unbelievable!

I shared with Uncle Butch my concerns over even owning a credit card. I had heard countless horror tales for years resulting from the serious issues they can create. He agreed that conventional wisdom does indeed suggest that young people should not own credit cards because of the dangers of debt, overspending, exorbitant finance charges, and destroying their credit scores after defaulting on a payment. He said that my fear was well-founded for 90 percent of people but not for the ten percent who are smart and responsible. He would show me how to qualify to be among the ten percent.

He explained that I am to charge every purchase from a hot dog to a computer using the bank's money free for 30 or 31 days each month. On the last day of the month, I am to pay in full the balance charged. In effect, I only use my money 12 days a year and the bank's money 353 days free of interest charges or fees.

As a bonus to me for using the bank's "free" money, they will pay me 3% cash back in a category of my choice, 2% cashback at grocery stores and wholesale clubs, and unlimited 1% cash back on all other purchases (on the first $2,500 in combined purchases each quarter)

Therefore, following Uncle Butch's ingenious plan, the monthly cash back rewards are deposited in my bank account, then transferred to my stock account. Accordingly, I can purchase a proportionate amount of positions in my S & P 500 Index fund.

In summary terms, the bank issued me a cost-free credit card that allows me to use interest-free money all but 12 days a year and pays me to use their money. The only condition is I must pay off the monthly statement in total each month without exception; otherwise, I will be paying over 20% interest on the unpaid balance—a formula for doom and the very reason 90% of folks should never own a credit card.

By maintaining a zero balance at the beginning of each month, I build my credit score rating for future larger purchases with each month's payment. The stocks will pay my account dividends automatically to purchase more stocks every three months. As I dollar-cost average additional purchases within my Roth Retirement account, I am off to the races securing my financial future, as uncle Butch termed it.

As a new employee at the beginning of my earnings cycles, my cash back rewards will be at the lowest levels. However, as I build up the total balances of all my bank's accounts—checking, cds, money markets, savings, and stocks—I can qualify to receive preferred rewards bonuses from 25%-75%. In time, these bonuses added to the base percentage can produce returns as high as 5.25% every quarter (3%+2.5%.) under current Federal Reserve monetary policies.

Consequently, it is plausible for me to receive $525.00 a year in cash rewards—enough to purchase two additional positions in my Roth S & P index fund of 500 stocks. How could a bank and credit card company possibly stay in business lending money for free and paying people to use their free money? Because human nature has proven, people tend to be undisciplined, and as high as 90% do not pay up at the end of the month. The lenders lose in this deal to the 10% of disciplined people, but are willing to do it because they do quite well with the projected 90% continuing debtors paying 20% interest each month—a foolish use of credit.

Uncle Butch changed my mind about owning credit cards, especially for the 10% of responsible people who use the banks' money for free and get paid to use it. I continue to use the "0" annual fee card he gave me, which pays rewards on all purchases with which I charge everything and pay the statement in full at the end of each month. I take my rewards in cash and invest it in a Roth S & P 500 Index Fund which returned year to date 13.8% interest. Compared to bank savings accounts at 0.05 %, the fund would double in 5.2 years whereas the current bank interest would take 1,440 to double.

Free online university classes - Over 900 of them provide free courses online. They include Oxford in England, the world's oldest English university, along with top-ranked Harvard. The Massachusetts Institute of Technology (MIT), Cal-tech, and Stanford. Harvard alone offers over 600. My grandfather is enrolled in their online studies and perhaps is their oldest student at 85!
www.coursera.org links to 200 universities and companies offering 4,777 courses. I recommend the free course "Measuring and maximizing the impact of COVID-19." Contact Johns Hopkins University at hub.jhu.edu.

The preceding activities are not exhaustive in context with the many suggestions I received from my family, friends, and unique resources. I have featured the ones that best refocused my attention away from the doom and gloom I experienced during my quarantine. I became utterly enthralled in playing, learning, and growing due to the ill wind, COVID-19, that ironically blew me some good and hopefully will for others...

The Rest of the Story

As the famous Paul Harvey from my parent's era signed off his radio show each day, "and now you [should] know, the rest of the story."

- ▶ July 2, 2020, I was cleared from quarantine and able to return to work.
- ▶ July 10, 2020, I took the NCLEX-RN exam. The National Council Licensure Examination was given to determine if it was safe for me to begin practice as an entry-level nurse.
- ▶ July 11, 2020, I learned that I passed the NCLEX-RN examination.
- ▶ July 16, 2020, I donated my plasma containing positive antibodies to combat the COVID-19 virus. I have heard from the Red Cross that it was used four times as a life-saving procedure for other patients.
- ▶ August 1, 2020, was my first shift as a Registered Nurse.
- ▶ November 9, 2020- Pfizer Pharmaceuticals and its German partner Biotech have developed a vaccine that is 90% effective in preventing infection from COVID-19. The impact remains to be seen.
- ▶ Global Status Report as of November 10, 2020
  Total cases–50,994,215 (rapidly increasing daily)
  Deaths–1,264,177 worldwide and 238,251 in the USA
- ▶ November 16, 2020, Moderna Pharmaceuticals followed Pfizer with a vaccine that reduced the risk of COVID-19 infection by 94.5%.
- ▶ November 23, 2020, the BioPharmaceutical Company, AstraZeneca, added another coronavirus vaccine to the mix, although it was only 70% effective.

Statistics Update as of 11/23/2020

Global status
58,766,000 cases

Deaths
Worldwide 1,389,000
U.S. 256,782 [68]

Encouraging news is breaking daily, including White House predictions that life could return to normal by May 2021!

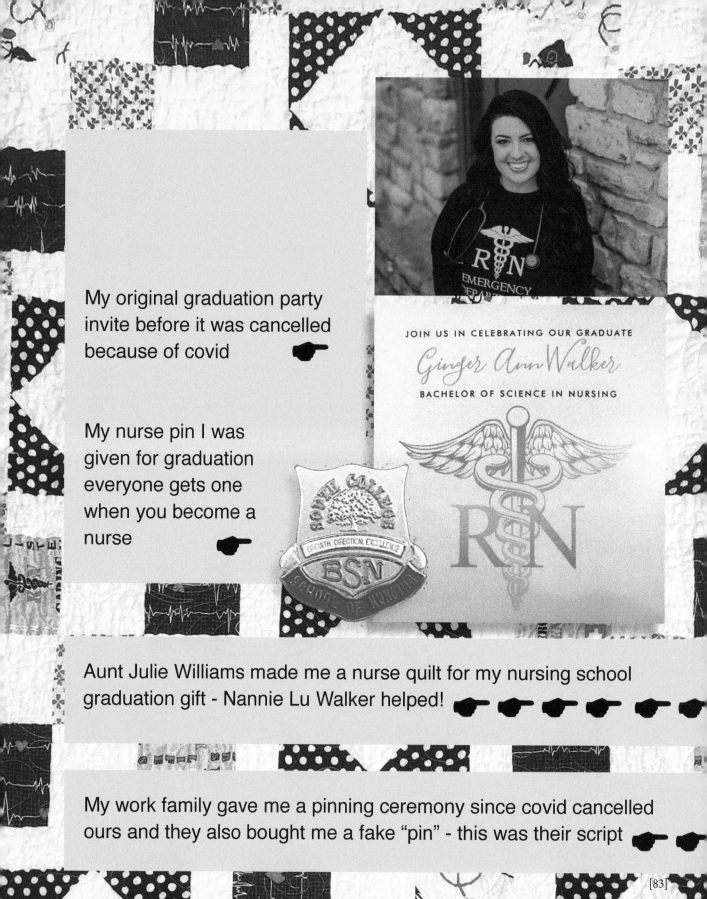

My original graduation party invite before it was cancelled because of covid 👉

My nurse pin I was given for graduation everyone gets one when you become a nurse 👉

JOIN US IN CELEBRATING OUR GRADUATE

Ginger Ann Walker

BACHELOR OF SCIENCE IN NURSING

RN

Aunt Julie Williams made me a nurse quilt for my nursing school graduation gift - Nannie Lu Walker helped! 👉 👉 👉 👉 👉 👉

My work family gave me a pinning ceremony since covid cancelled ours and they also bought me a fake "pin" - this was their script 👉 👉

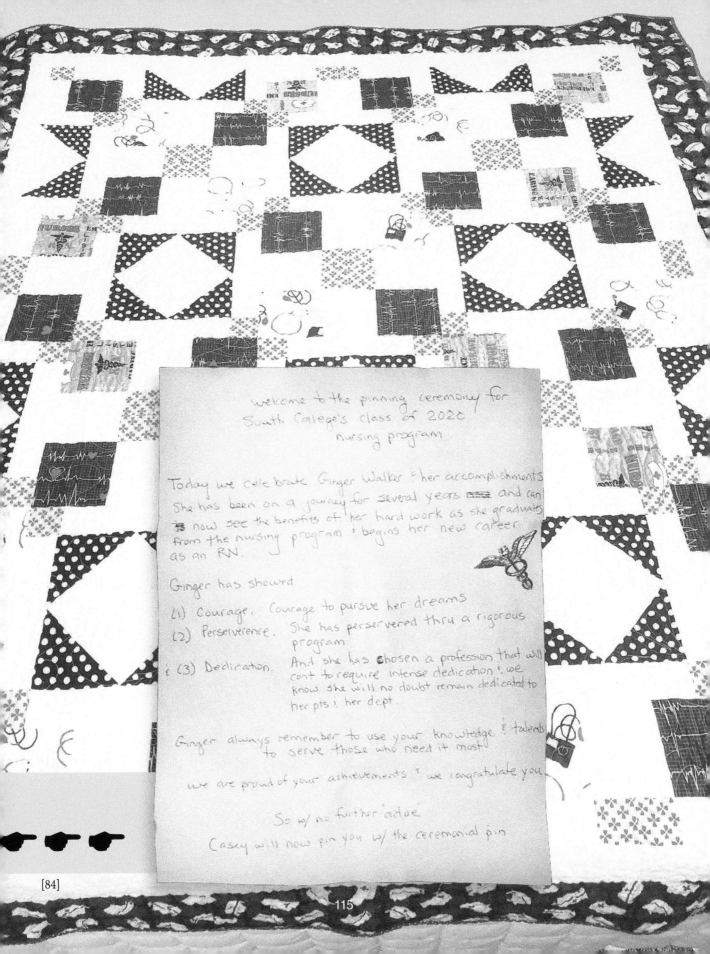

welcome to the pinning ceremony for
South College's class of 2020
nursing program

Today we celebrate Ginger Walker & her accomplishments.
She has been on a journey for several years and can
now see the benefits of her hard work as she graduates
from the nursing program & begins her new career
as an RN.

Ginger has showed

(1) Courage. Courage to pursue her dreams

(2) Perserverence. She has perservered thru a rigorous
program

& (3) Dedication. And she has chosen a profession that will
cont to require intense dedication & we
know she will no doubt remain dedicated to
her pts & her dept.

Ginger always remember to use your knowledge & talents
to serve those who need it most!

we are proud of your achievements & we congratulate you.

So w/ no further adue

Casey will now pin you w/ the ceremonial pin

VALEDICTION

It was June 5th, 2020, when I was diagnosed with the COVID-19 virus. It has taken approximately six-months for me to transcend from the negative impact of this infectious disease to several positive outcomes.

The highlight came from the American Red Cross, telling me that my donated plasma was utilized to save lives and provide research to find a treatment and cure for future patients.

The isolation factor created from being quarantined for a month forced me to become a more rounded person and motivated learner in several domains. Frankly, I never felt a desire to acquire knowledge, skills, and competencies beyond a specific job requirement. The continually changing paradigm caused by the current pandemic and the horrifying punishment of solitary confinement forced me to change my thinking and behavior.

I learned directly that fear and love are the two most powerful motivators of behavior, but they cannot coexist. In my faith, the Epistle of Jude addresses the influences that stir people to action; it asserts that compassion achieves nobler and more enduring results than fear. I discovered the truth of this in a newly found love for learning and especially from the shared experiences of the older and wiser "who know they know." I hasten to admit that in my early years, I thought I knew it all—more than my parents, teachers, preachers, the world, but when introduced to COVID-19, I discovered "I knew not."

"HE WHO KNOWS NOT, AND KNOWS NOT THAT HE KNOWS NOT,
 IS A FOOL; SHUN HIM.

HE WHO KNOWS NOT, AND KNOWS THAT HE KNOWS NOT,
 IS A STUDENT; TEACH HIM.

He who knows, and knows not that he knows,
is asleep; wake him.

He who knows, and knows that he knows, is wise;
follow him."[69]

— Arabian Proverb

My mission in this effort has been to provide real-time, eye-witness COVID-19 information to those who are infected, may become infected, are attempting to avoid infection, or are serving those who are infected. This group includes research scientists, doctors, nurses, patients, students, family members, and the general public. My daily experiences and studies have provided the narrative.

Now that you have seen my story in real-time, it is my sincere hope that you have found the content to be of redeeming value. My prayer especially is that the message and examples help fill voids in the minds, bodies, and spirits of the lonely—patients and otherwise.

To all caregivers and medical professionals addressing COVID-19 patients in your charge: Until a 100% effective vaccine is developed, your prescribed protocols and regimens must include ways and means of combatting the physical and mental damage caused by solitary confinement. I found this to be the major adversary lurking within the disease but far more sinister. Hopefully, I have given you food for thought.

Thank you for reading and considering.

Best wishes,

Dinger

"I wandered lonely as a cloud that floats on high o'er vales and hills

...for oft, when on my couch I lie

...in pensive mood,

...which is the bliss of solitude;

and then my heart

with pleasure fills..."[70]

I Wandered Lonely as a Cloud—William Wordsworth.

EPILOGUE

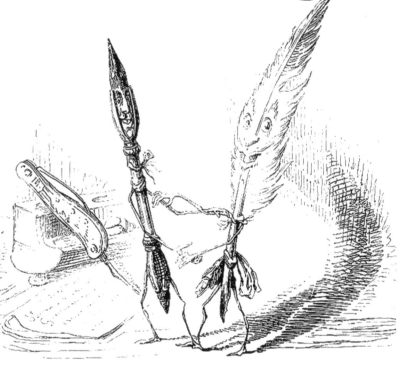

[85] *Autre Monde Epilog* by J.J. Grandville

During my isolation, I grew to appreciate Surrealism. This unusual art style captures one's imagination while granting boundless interpretations. Surrealist J.J. Grandville illustrates here in his *Un Autre Monde Epilog* a subtle parallel to my Epilogue, which is an afterword to the latest developments in search of a treatment and cure for Covid-19.

His illustration above personifies an argument between a pen and a pencil—neither chooses to seize the nearby knife to gain an advantage or risk further escalation. As an alternative, the combatants stopped fighting. They agreed in the illustration on the right that Un Autre Monde (a different world or way) is masterful—the best possible epilogue to conflict. Each is given a platform and can function peacefully as an artist and a writer without being enemies.

The example suggests that without compelling evidence, the most practical path is not to assume Covid-19 was created and spread intentionally but to focus on the treatment and cure. However, this conciliatory approach does not dismiss the possibility that a bioweapon was being produced and accidentally released, ultimately causing the current pandemic. There is whistleblower evidence that supports that conclusion. Throughout history, germ warfare inhumanely has been used to gain an advantage over enemies. Their use was outlawed in 1972 by the Biological Weapons Convention. However, John Lyly predicted the unlikelihood of compliance in his lines, "all is fair in love and war."

This last episode in my story was opened on January 14, 2021. Thirteen virus specialists representing the World Health Organization landed in Wuhan, China, where Covid-19 first was detected. They were from Australia, Britain, Germany, Japan, the Netherlands, Qatar, Russia, the United States, and Vietnam. After months of international wrangling, seeking to cast or deny blame, China President Xi Jinping has opened his doors to direct inquiry and examination.

The blame game has been a moving target and not productive. This virus has plunged the global economy into its most profound depression since the 1930s. To date, it has killed almost two million people since late 2019, and the number is growing daily exponentially. It remains to be seen if this WHO endeavor will confirm the origin of the virus or in the final analysis if it matters. The infected thousands of patients my universal family of coworkers and I admit to the world's emergency rooms each day are desperate. Please encourage and support them with your voice, purse, and pen.

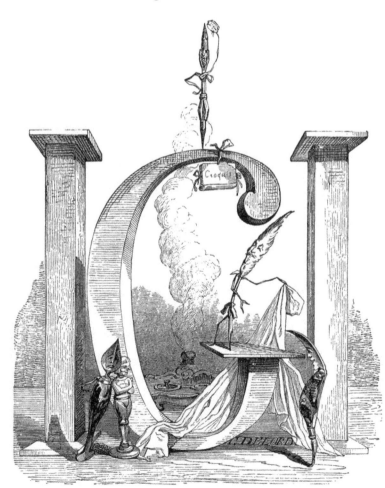

[86] *Fantastic-Illustrations-Grandville-Autre-Animax*

ABOUT THE CONTRIBUTORS

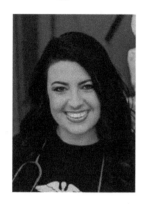

Author—Ginger Ann Walker The first assignment in this project came from my primary mentors, Great Aunt Nancy Arnold, and my Grandad, Ed Garrett. They asked me to introduce myself. As the readers can see from what author Jack Van Hooser wrote about them, I have been under the guidance of experienced professionals in this, my first writing venture. They modestly make no such claims, but their self-publishing accomplishments spanning four continents are significant.

Regarding my writing assignment, I was born at Baptist Hospital in Nashville, Tennessee, on October 14, 1996. Coincidentally, I am employed just a short elevator ride to the floor and ward where I was born.

I attended Rutland Elementary School in Wilson County, Tennessee, where my mother was a teacher, as another coincidence. The middle school years were at West Wilson Middle, and subsequently, I graduated from Wilson Central High School in 2015.

I was reared in a Christian home and professed my Faith accordingly at my age of accountability.

My first regular job was at Courtney's Restaurant in Mt. Juliet, Tennessee, the homes of the famed Charlie Daniels and master fisherman, Coach Rees Groce—who taught me how to catch crappie. I am grateful to Tom Courtney for hiring a fledgling teenager and reinforcing the strong work ethic ingrained by my father, Mike Walker.

This early grounding helped make me want to choose a career with a mission and purpose of helping people, but I did not know it would be in nursing. As I began to take science classes in high school, I became increasingly interested in anatomy and physiology and how the human body functions. Later, that led me to become certified as a nurse assistant-CNA, which enabled me to work in a nursing home. As time elapsed, I became convinced that becoming a Registered Nurse was my choice and perhaps calling. I enrolled in South College and began my journey. The rest of the story you already have read or will follow.

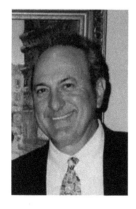

Editor—Garrett Williams, a.k.a. John "Ed" Garrett (Ginger's grandfather)

Ginger's Granddad was born and nurtured in Springfield, Tennessee, and has lived most of his adult years in the Madison Community of Metropolitan Nashville and Davidson County, Tennessee. He was a four-decade career educator with the Metro Public School District as a classroom teacher, supervisor, and H.R. Director for the Secondary Schools. He married his high school sweetheart, Ginger's grandmother, the former Jo Ann Adams, and they have two children and six grandchildren.

Ed's talents beyond the classroom have awarded him U.S. patents and copyrights for intellectual property creations, including a public television media production, two personal books, and ghost writings resulting in four additional published books and several magazine articles. His first authorship was on behalf of the famous guitarist brothers Chet and Jim Atkins. They utilized Ed's skills to write the **Famous American Musicians and Educators** teacher's manual. Subsequently, **Misguided Notions** was his treatise about 10,000 years of educational history. Thereafter, Ed collaborated with Ed (Hanes) to produce **The Little Evergreen's Dream**, a popular early intervention resource enabling parents and teachers to guide young children in matters related to bullying. Prior to **COVID-19 In Real-Time**, he co-authored **Old Glory—From Salem to Nashville, The Life and Times of Patriot William Driver.**

Ed's pseudonym as a writer is Garrett Williams in honor of his father and mother. I have known him in diverse roles for over 50 years. I have utilized his knowledge and skills and those of the forthcoming Nancy Arnold in publishing two books, **A Journey to Remember** and **Unstable Times-Unlikely Outcomes**. With admiration, I call him a "wordsmith." You will enjoy his creative contributions to his granddaughter's COVID-19 book. —Jack Van Hooser - author

Graphic Design and Production—Nancy Adams Arnold

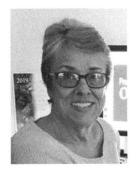

Nancy's artistic gifts and creative talents became apparent to all observers during her pre-teen years in Cedar Hill, Tennessee. She utilized nature and country life as her studio for drawing, painting, and photography. At age 12, formal lessons began, followed by teacher recommended summer employment preparing art for silk-screening. Next were stints with the Newspaper Printing Corporation, Design Graphics, Inc., and the Baptist Sunday School Board facilitating ad and mechanical layouts and preparing camera-ready art.

Her horizons continued to broaden through the years as the printing process changed from hot metal to computer-generated page layout and various experiences, including a trip to Rome and the Holy Land, leading to photography specialization for religious publications. She worked at BSSB, now LifeWay Christian Resources, for 17 years full-time and freelance for a total of 40 years.

Nancy lives in Springfield, Tennessee, with husband Eddie and Lucky, everyone's favorite Chihuahua. She is a proud mom of two children, grandma to four, and great-grandma to four more. She enjoys using her skills "to play" in Photoshop and InDesign, retouch old photographs, helping others self-publish books, designing brochures, genealogical research, and other special projects.

Along with this current publication about Ginger Ann Walker's encounter with COVID 19 and **Old Glory From Salem to Nashville, the Life and Times of William Driver,** I invite readers to examine her excellent visuals and layouts found in my two above referenced books. —Jack Van Hooser - author

RESOURCES

Page-Citation

iv   1 https://www.goodreads.com/author/show/229.Abraham_Lincoln (accessed 10-19-2020)

iv   2 https://www.nps.gov/mlkm/learn/quotations.htm#:~:text=%22The%20ultimate%20measure%20of%20a,best%20in%20 their%20individual%20societies.%22 (Accessed 10-19-2020)

3   3 https://en.wikipedia.org/wiki/In_Color_(song)(Accessed 10-19-2020)

4   4 https://www.fda.gov/news-events/press-announcements/coronavirus-covid-19-update-fda-authorizes-first-test-detects-neutralizing-antibodies-recent-or (Accessed 10-19-2020)

12   5 https://www.who.int/docs/default-source/coronaviruse/situation-reports/20200121-sitrep-1-2019-ncov.pdf (Accessed 10-19-2020)

12   6 https://www.seattletimes.com/seattle-news/health/case-of-wuhan-coronavirus-detected-in-washington-state-first-in-united-states/ (Accessed 10-20-2020)

14   7 https://en.wikipedia.org/wiki/Li-Meng_Yan (Accessed 10-19-2020)

15   8 https://www.animalsasia.org/us/our-work/cat-and-dog-welfare/facts-about-dog-meat-trade.html (Accessed 10-19-2020)

15   9 https://www.ncbi.nlm.nih.gov/pmc/articles/PMC3291347/ (Accessed 10-19-2020)

18   10 https://www.cdc.gov/coronavirus/2019-ncov/symptoms-testing/symptoms.html (Accessed (10-19-2020)

19   11 https://www.cnn.com/2019/09/25/health/best-drinks-for-hydration-wellness/index.html (Accessed 10-19-2020)

20   11a https://en.wikipedia.org/wiki/Energy_drink (Accessed-10-19-2020)

20   11b https://nutrition.ucdavis.edu/outreach/nutr-health-info-sheets/pro-caffeine (Accessed-10-19-2020)

20   12 https://www.samhsa.gov/data/sites/default/files/spot124-energy-drinks-2014.pdf (Accessed 10-19-2020)

21   12a https://www.hsph.harvard.edu/nutritionsource/energy-drinks/ (Accessed-10-19-2020)

21   13 https://www.nationalacademies.org/news/2004/02/report-sets-dietary-intake-levels-for-water-salt-and-potassium-to-maintain-health-and-reduce-chronic-disease-risk (Accessed 10-19-2020)

22   14 https://www.smithsonianmag.com/smart-news/america-has-been-struggling-metric-system-almost-230-years-180964147/ (Accessed 10-19-2020)

23   15 https://drinkbiolyte.com/ (Accessed 10-19-2020)

29   16 https://en.wikipedia.org/wiki/I_Can_See_Clearly_Now (Accessed 10-19-2020)

31   16a https://www.hsph.harvard.edu/news/hsph-in-the-news/covid-19-vaccines-unlikely-to-be-cure-all/ (Accessed-10-19-2020)

32   17 https://www.alice-in-wonderland.net/ (Accessed 10-19-2020)

32   18 https://en.wikipedia.org/wiki/Dale_Carnegie (Accessed 10-19-2020)

34   18a https://www.medicinanarrativa.eu/so-much-inside-alice-wonderland-for-medical-humanities (Accessed-10-19-2020)

35   18b https://news.un.org/en/story/2011/10/392012-solitary-confinement-should-be-banned- (Accessed-10-19-2020)

35   19 https://en.wikipedia.org/wiki/To_Althea,_from_Prison (Accessed 10-19-2020)

36   20 https://academic.oup.com/qjmed/article/113/8/527/5860844 (Accessed 10-19-2020)

37   21 https://www.theloop.ca/alice-in-wonderland-nasa-and-einstein-all-have-something-very-strange-in-common/ (Accessed 10-19-2020)

37   22 https://www.biography.com/news/albert-einstein-iq (Accessed 10-19-2020)

40   23 https://www.alsintl.com/poetry/thehousebythesideoftheroad.htm (Accessed 10-19-2020)

41   24 https://plato.stanford.edu/entries/ockham/ (Accessed 10-19-2020)

42   25 https://www.rubegoldberg.com/the-man-behind-the-machine/ (Accessed 10-19-2020)

47   26 https://www.goodreads.com/quotes/7-it-is-not-the-critic-who-counts-not-the-man https://www.poetryfoundation.org/poems/48860/the-raven (Accessed-10-19-2020)

48   27 https://www.wealthwords.com/blog/author/nikitab/ (Accessed 10-19-2020)

52   28 https://www.healthline.com/health/benefits-of-reading-books (Accessed 10-19-2020)

53   29 https://susanwisebauer.com/the-well-educated-mind-a-guide-to-the-classical-education-you-never-had/ (Accessed 10-19-2020)

57   30 https://en.wikipedia.org/wiki/Evelyn_Wood_(teacher) (Accessed 10-19-2020)

58 31 https://www.goodreads.com/quotes/408441-a-reader-lives-a-thousand-lives-before-he-dies-said (Accessed 10-19-2020)

59 32 https://en.wikipedia.org/wiki/Little_Things_Mean_a_Lot (Accessed 10-19-2020)

60 33 https://www.brainyquote.com/quotes/yehuda_berg_536651https://www.brainyquote.com/quotes/yehuda_berg_536651 (Accessed 10-19-2020)

62 34 https://archive.org/stream/AnthonyRobbinsUnlimitedPower/Anthony%20Robbins%20Unlimited%20Power_djvu.txt (Accessed 10-19-2020)

63 35 https://www.scientificamerican.com/article/do-people-only-use-10-percent-of-their-brains/ (Accessed 10-19-2020)

63 36 https://med.stanford.edu/news/all-news/2010/11/new-imaging-method-developed-at-stanford-reveals-stunning-details-of-brain-connections.html (Accessed 10-19-2020)

63 37 https://www.cnsnevada.com/what-is-the-memory-capacity-of-a-human-brain/https://www.eurekalert.org/pub_releases/2020-10/f-mtc100220.php (Accessed 10-19-2020)

64 38 https://www.poetryfoundation.org/poems/48860/the-ravenhttps://www.poetryfoundation.org/poems/48860/the-raven (Accessed 10-19-2020)

65 39 https://www.npr.org/sections/thetwo-way/2009/12/poe_book_auctioned_for_662500.html (Accessed 10-19-2020)

66 40 https://classicalpoets.org/2016/01/07/10-greatest-poems-ever-written/ (Accessed 10-19-2020)

66 41 https://www.psychologytoday.com/us/blog/memory-medic/201305/memorization-is-not-dirty-word-2 (Accessed 10-19-2020)

67 42 https://www.eurekalert.org/pub_releases/2020-10/f-mtc100220.php (Accessed 10-19-2020)

68 43 https://www.newsweek.com/spotify-reveals-music-surgeons-love-listening-operating-room-645322 (Accessed 10-19-2020)

68 44 https://theconversation.com/whether-mozart-or-madonna-music-can-help-you-recover-from-surgery-45973 (Accessed 10-19-2020)

68 45 https://brainupfl.org/2019/11/09/memorizing-is-a-lost-art-but-should-it-be/ (Accessed 10-19-2020)

71 46 https://www.nytimes.com/interactive/2020/10/05/science/charting-a-covid-immune-response.html (Accessed 10-19-2020)

73 47 https://www.goodreads.com/quotes/4673-art-washes-away-from-the-soul-the-dust-of-everyday (Accessed 10-19-2020)

74 48 https://www.colonialflag.com/symbolism-of-the-red-white-and-blue/ (Accessed 10-19-2020)

74 49 https://en.wikipedia.org/wiki/Bob_Dole (Accessed 10-19-2020)

75 50 https://www.wideopencountry.com/billy-ray-cyrus-some-gave-all/ (Accessed 10-19-2020)

77 51 https://amhistory.si.edu/starspangledbanner/the-lyrics.aspx (Accessed 10-19-2020)

78 52 https://www.verywellmind.com/elizabeth-scott-m-s-3144382 (Accessed 10-19-2020)

81 53 https://www.animallaw.info/article/faqs-emotional-support-animals (Accessed 10-19-2020)

84 54 https://www.health.harvard.edu/mind-and-mood/how-meditation-helps-with-depression (Accessed 10-19-2020)

85 55 https://www.hinduismtoday.com/modules/smartsection/item.php?itemid=1456 (Accessed 10-19-2020)

85 56 https://my.clevelandclinic.org/health/articles/16779-aerobic-exercise--heart-health (Accessed 10-19-2020)

85 57 https://www.cbsnews.com/news/movie-therapy-using-movies-for-mental-health/ (Accessed 10-19-2020)

89 58 https://news.uga.edu/feeling-depressed-mahjong-might-be-answer/ (Accessed 10-19-2020)

90 59 https://www.fractuslearning.com/some-surprising-benefits-of-lego/ (Accessed 10-19-2020)

91 60 https://www.archives.gov/files/research/census/ (Accessed 10-19-2020)

95 61 https://en.wikipedia.org/wiki/Far_Away_Places (Accessed 10-19-2020)

95 62 https://www.ancient.eu/Byzantine_Empire/ (Accessed 10-19-2020)

97 63 https://en.wikipedia.org/wiki/Fall_of_Constantinople (Accessed 10-19-2020)

97 64 https://turkeytravelplanner.com/Religion/index.html (Accessed 10-19-2020)

98 65 https://en.wikipedia.org/wiki/Major_religious_groups (Accessed 10-19-2020)

101 66 https://theroamingrenegades.com/blue-mosque-hagia-sophia-istanbul/ (Accessed 10-19-2020)

106 67 https://finance.zacks.com/new-york-stock-exchange-largest-stock-market-world-5426.html (Accessed 10-19-2020)

113 68 https://www.patientcareonline.com/view/covid-19-update-us-and-global-cases-deaths-and-recoveries-as-of-november-23-2020 (Accessed 10-19-2020)

116 69 https://en.wikipedia.org/wiki/I_know_that_I_know_nothing (Accessed 11-5-2020)

119 70 https://en.wikisource.org/wiki/I_Wandered_Lonely_as_a_Cloud (Accessed 11-5-2020)

Page-Image

67 [44] https://en.wikipedia.org/wiki/Thriller_(album) (Accessed 10-19-2020)

69 [45] https://collections.artsmia.org/art/54270/david-playing-the-harp-before-saul-lucas-huygensz-van-leyden (Accessed 10-19-2020)

70 [46] https://en.wikipedia.org/wiki/Quill (Accessed 10-19-2020)

72 [47] https://en.wikipedia.org/wiki/COVID-19_vaccine (Accessed 10-19-2020)

73 [48] https://en.wikipedia.org/wiki/File:Pablo_Picasso,_1902- 3,Femme_assise_(Melancholy_Woman),_oil_on_canvas,_100_x_69.2_ cm,_ (Accessed 10-19-2020)

75 [49] https://doyouremember.com/88923/bob-dole-salutes-bush-casket (Accessed 10-19-2020)

76 [50] *I stand for the Nation Anthem* by Ed Garrett

77 [50a] Photo by Ed Garrett

77 [51] *Old Glory* by Jack Benz and Garrett Williams

77 [52] *Old Glory Abridged* by Jack Benz and Garrett Williams

78 [53] https://en.wikipedia.org/wiki/Emotion_in_animals (Accessed 10-19-2020)

79 [54] Knoxville by Ginger Walker

80 [55] Knoxville by Ginger Walker

80 [56] Knoxville by Ginger Walker

80 [57] Family collectable John Garrett

81 [58] Family Christmas by Carol Blackmon

82 [59] by Nancy Arnold

83 [60] by Ed Garrett public domain images (Accessed 10-19-2020)

84 [61] https://www.stylecraze.com/articles/dhyana-yoga-what-is-it-and-what-are-its-benefits/ (Accessed 10-19-2020)

86 [62] https://en.wikipedia.org/wiki/Gone_with_the_Wind_(film) (Accessed 10-19-2020)

89 [63] https://en.wikipedia.org/wiki/Klondike_(solitaire) (Accessed 10-19-2020)

89 [64] https://en.wikipedia.org/wiki/Mahjong_solitaire (Accessed 10-19-2020)

89 [65] https://en.wikipedia.org/https://upload.wikimedia.org/wikipedia/commons/0/0f/2_duplo_lego_bricks.jpg? (Accessed 10-19-2020)

92 [66] https://upload.wikimedia.org/wikipedia/commons/f/fa/Globe.svg (Accessed 10-19-2020)

94 [67] https://en.wikipedia.org/wiki/Geography_of_Panama#/media/File:Pm-map.png (Accessed 10-19-2020)

95 [68] https://commons.wikimedia.org/wiki/File:Turkey-CIA_WFB_Map.png (Accessed 10-19-2020)

96 [69] https://commons.wikimedia.org/wiki/File:Hagia_Sophia_2.jpg (Accessed 10-19-2020)

97 [70] https://en.wikipedia.org/wiki/Sujud (Accessed 10-19-2020)

98 [71] https://en.wikipedia.org/wiki/Star_and_crescent (Accessed 10-19-2020)

99 [72] https://en.wikipedia.org/wiki/Aqueduct_of_Valens (Accessed 10-19-2020)

100 [73] https://en.wikipedia.org/wiki/Grand_Bazaar,_Istanbul (Accessed 10-19-2020)

100 [74] https://en.wikipedia.org/wiki/Turkish_bath (Accessed 10-19-2020)

101 [75] https://en.wikipedia.org/wiki/Sultan_Ahmed_Mosque (Accessed 10-19-2020)

101 [76] https://en.wikipedia.org/wiki/Sultan_Ahmed_Mosque#/media/File:Inside_Blue_Mosque_3.jpg (Accessed 10-19-2020)

102 [77] https://en.wikipedia.org/wiki/Kebab (Accessed 10-19-2020)

103 [78] https://en.wikipedia.org/wiki/Dondurma#/media/File:Dondurma_(5065600007).jpg (Accessed 10-19-2020)

104 [79] Law of Compounding by Nancy Arnold

105 [80] http://www.cathedralguadalupe.org/bulletin/2014/111614.pdf (Accessed 10-19-2020)

107 [81] https://commons.wikimedia.org/wiki/File:S_and_P_500_chart_1950_to_2016_with_averages.png (Accessed 10-19-2020)

109 [82] Question Mark crafted by Nancy Arnold

114 [83] Collage crafted by Nancy Arnold

115 [84] Collage crafted by Nancy Arnold

120 [85] https://upload.wikimedia.org/wikipedia/commons/0/07/Grandville%2C_Autre_Monde%2C_Epilog.jpg (Accessed 1-9-2020)

121 [86] *Fantastic-Illustrations-Grandville-Autre-Animax*/dp/0486229912 permission Garrett Williams